ETHICAL ISSUES IN THE 21ST CENTURY

PATIENT RIGHTS

ETHICAL PERSPECTIVES, EMERGING DEVELOPMENTS AND GLOBAL CHALLENGES

ETHICAL ISSUES IN THE 21ST CENTURY

Additional books in this series can be found on Nova's website under the Series tab.

Additional e-books in this series can be found on Nova's website under the e-book tab.

ETHICAL ISSUES IN THE 21ST CENTURY E

PATIENT RIGHTS

ETHICAL PERSPECTIVES, EMERGING DEVELOPMENTS AND GLOBAL CHALLENGES

JENNA POPE
EDITOR

nova publishers
New York

Library of Congress Cataloging-in-Publication Data

ISBN: 978-1-63482-136-0

Published by Nova Science Publishers, Inc. † New York

CONTENTS

PREFACE

In the past 50 years, ethical concerns concerning human experimentation have arisen with the advancement of new medical research and technology. While the benefits of human experimentation are well known in the fields of biology, psychology, sociology, and medicine, the conditions of human subject research have been persistently controversial. This book discusses ethical perspectives, emerging developments and global challenged of patient rights. Topics include effective medical informed consent; rights to health and dental care; the ethics of HIV screening targeted to the seriously mentally ill; and problems in ethics for medical publication.

Chapter 1 – Traditional healthcare ethics has flourished in an environment of ethical principlism, with its focus on patient privacy and autonomy. Clinical genetic testing and tissue banking utilize protocols that rest on a combination of autonomy and beneficence, incorporated into codes of professional practice. Exceptions occur under a case-based rubric, but these departures are the minority. Public health, with its emphasis on the common good and general welfare of the greater population, invokes additional ethical-legal features such as the "*parens patriae*" doctrine and a spectrum of means to assure health that go beyond traditional consent. This protective legal blanket moves solidaristic and communitarian principles to the forefront. In our chapter the authors look at significant new developments in the genomics field – family risk assessment (using family health history and cascade genetic screening) and population biobanking. The authors describe new forms of consent that have arisen in response to group-level genetic interventions, as well as the conflicts and compromises that arise with institutional privacy rules. The shift towards a public health ethics calls for a form of synergistic ethics in which benefits to any one individual mutually enhance benefits to all in need. This enlarged ethical perspective aims at a concept of personalized risk assessment and management in the context of public, as opposed to strictly individual, health.

Chapter 2 – In the past 50 years, ethical concerns concerning human experimentation have arisen with the advancement of new medical research and technology. While the benefits of human experimentation are well known in the fields of biology, psychology, sociology, and medicine, the conditions of human subject research have been persistently controversial. Our current healthcare model operates based on a distinction between clinical care and clinical research. Subsequently, several bioethicists have argued that this segregated model poses several conceptual, moral and empirical problems. As a result, some have suggested blurring the line between clinical research and clinical care. One such plan to blur this line is by randomizing the type of therapy given to patients and collecting data from it if the treatment options have similar risk profiles. A potential problem with any new change in a system that monitors human subject research is the over- or under-protection of research subjects (patients in this case). In the authors' commentary, he will highlight four potential issues that he can foresee happening under the proposal of routinely randomizing medical interventions: [i] patients' health and well-being may be compromised, [ii] patients' preferences may not be respected, [iii] patients' privacy may be violated, and [iv] physicians' judgment may be restricted. To prevent these four problems, the author proposes that we fulfill four criteria that are aimed to prevent the over- or under-protection of research subjects under a randomization proposal.

Chapter 3 – Few would disagree with the desirability of patients providing informed consent before undergoing medical treatments. However, the authors believe that the obstacles to this goal are more numerous and difficult than bioethicists have realized. Even under ideal circumstances where doctors provide all of the relevant information, a variety of patient limitations may prevent them from using the information properly; in short, patients might be unable to provide *effective* informed consent. In addition, a variety of factors might prevent doctors from providing all of the relevant information in a way that patients can use, or even in any form whatsoever. Finally, the authors argue that the courts (appropriately) have set legal standards that are lower than ideal bioethical standards, and so legal considerations are capable of providing only the smallest of pushes in the direction of ethical behavior. The authors challenge the bioethical community to find solutions to all three categories of issues.

Chapter 4 – Complex mechanisms are in place to protect research subjects and to ensure that participants are informed of the risks, benefits, and alternatives available to them prior to enrolling in a research study. However, the process for obtaining informed consent is obscured in the setting of medical emergencies, specifically when subjects are incapacitated. This makes progress in emergency, trauma, and resuscitation research challenging, disciplines in which there is an ongoing need to improve diagnostic and management strategies. There are several guidelines—such as the Declaration of Helsinki, The Common Rule, and the Final Rule—to help researchers navigate this terrain. Unfortunately, none of these regulations sufficiently defines the nuances regarding informed consent among patients in need of emergent intervention. In this chapter, the authors seek to shed light on the ethical and regulatory considerations surrounding research subjects in emergent medical situations, particularly with regard to the appropriate interpretation of informed consent. As the administrative landscape continues to evolve, principles concerning emergency research should be further standardized to offer sufficient protection to study subjects, while permitting research efforts to proceed without excessive regulatory burden. Throughout this process, it will be crucial for researchers to understand the ethical principles that dictate policy among this uniquely vulnerable population.

Chapter 5 – Universal access to oral health care is a fundamental right for everyone and the primary purpose of all health care professionals, organizations, and public policy should be to improve oral health. In today's economic climate, health care systems are challenged by the need to prioritise and address the inequitable distribution of resources in society. Market forces, scarcity of funding, and lack of clarity as to who is responsible for ensuring that oral care is available add to these difficulties. Dentistry is not part of the universal health care system in all countries: inequalities within dentistry are common and reflected in wide differences in the levels of oral health and the standard of care available both within and between countries and communities. Oral health care is complex and there is no consensus within the profession about what counts as normal human functioning and little consensus about what basic needs entail especially where resources are limited. Moreover, vulnerable populations are often further disadvantaged by physical disabilities, illness, poverty, and other socio-economic conditions that impede their access to care. Improving access to oral health care is a social problem intimately intertwined with general health care access, education, and oral health literacy of the public, employment, insurance, and a host of other societal factors. The dental professions will not solve these problems in isolation: a systematic approach is essential if we are to understand, evaluate, and institute structural, organizational, professional, and individual change in the oral health delivery system.

Chapter 6 – *Background:* There is a higher than expected global prevalence of HIV risk behavior among adults with severe mental illness (SMI) and a consequently high HIV prevalence. The US Center for Disease Control recommends yearly HIV testing of high-risk groups but the SMI population is rarely tested. Objective: This chapter discusses the pros and cons of provider-initiated screening for HIV in mental health settings that serve the seriously mentally ill. *Method:* A literature review of the ethics of HIV screening as it pertains to the seriously mentally ill. *Results:* There are several benefits to provider-initiated HIV screening of SMI patients in mental health settings. It motivates risk reduction behavior when accompanied by pretest and posttest counseling. Individuals who test positive obtain immediate access to ongoing medical care for HIV. The public health benefit is that at risk individuals modify their behavior and thus reduce incidence rates while HIV+ individuals obtain treatment that renders them less infectious, further driving down infection rates. There are ethical issues, however, that need to be addressed. Does targeting SMI individuals increase their stigmatization? Can provider-initiated screening be considered voluntary? Is consent in this cognitively challenged population truly informed? Do perceived incentives negate the voluntary aspect of consent? Can confidentiality be guaranteed in a mental health setting where service users constantly interact? Whose responsibility is it if HIV+ persons fail to disclose their status to sexual partners or fail to reduce risk behaviors? Does the public health benefit outweigh individual benefit? Is there a financial cost benefit? *Conclusion:* Ethical issues are important to consider and discuss. Safeguards need to be in place. On the whole, however, this paper endorses the provision of HIV screening in mental health settings for the seriously mentally ill.

Chapter 7 – Physicians generally accept two major reasons for nontruthful disclosure of information to patients even when the patients can make autonomous decisions: promoting the patients' best interests and preserving their autonomy. If physicians deceive or withhold information from such patients based on the first reason, the physicians act from paternalism. However, autonomous individuals are in the best position to determine their best interests. The manner in which patients understand their best interests may differ from the physician's perceptions; therefore, respecting patients' autonomy, rather than paternalistic practice, is the best way to promote patients' best interests. Nontruthful disclosure of information can be justified only when truth-telling will cause patients to lose their ability to make decisions reflecting their long-term values, i.e., only when truth-telling will compromise patients' autonomy. In general, paternalism is justified only when patients' autonomy has already been or is going to be compromised.

Chapter 8 – Medical publication is a common kind of literature in medical journals and books. Similar to any other kinds of science, the ethical problems in medical publication can be seen and it is an interesting issue in journalism. The misconducts in medical publication is of concern and the management is required. Here, the authors brief review and discussed on examples from Thailand.

Chapter 9 – The patient is the central figure in any healthcare system. In fact, she is the reason the system exists. In India, though the entire health care system has evolved around the patient, it is, strangely, the healer who is looked upon as the patron of the system. The doctor is positioned at the top of the social hierarchy while the patient is at the bottom, though the latter pays for everything. In the entire process, patients have few rights, and even those are limited to what the doctors deign to grant them. Doctors ensure that their authority never gets diluted. In case of disputes, medical colleagues support the doctor and not the patient. The patient is a helpless pawn in the game played by doctors, hospitals, laboratories and drug companies. Patients' rights are meant to protect them from these situations and any form of financial impropriety violates these rights. Unfortunately, financial impropriety in the medical world is a pervasive phenomenon, seen more often in developing countries where it is rampant throughout the hierarchy. This prevents the patients from having access to quality medical care. In India, the existing patients' rights provide no protection since the charter of rights is designed not to empower the patient, but to keep him in the power of the doctor. The average Indian survives many battles against health hazards caused by low quality water supply, poor sanitation, low standards of public health, high morbidity and mortality as well as indifference of doctors and administrators in the healthcare system. This leaves the citizens caught between a highly inefficient public health system and a largely unregulated and exploitive private health system. The physician, who is the final link to the patient, has the power to protect the patient, but more often than not, stands as a mute spectator. Patients here require more rights, especially those that will protect them against financial exploitation. They should also have the right to decide how they are treated in the terminal stages and should have the option to put in place directives that are legal and binding on families and attending physicians.

In: Patient Rights
Editor: Jenna Pope
ISBN: 978-1-63482-136-0

Chapter 1

DISTINCTIVE FEATURES OF PUBLIC HEALTH ETHICS IN THE DOMAIN OF EXPANDED GENETIC SCREENING AND POPULATION BIOBANKING

Stephen M. Modell[1,2], Toby Citrin[1], Jodyn E. Platt[1] and Sharon L. R. Kardia[2]
[1]Department of Health Management and Policy,
[2]Department of Epidemiology
University of Michigan School of Public Health,
Ann Arbor, MI, US

ABSTRACT

Traditional healthcare ethics has flourished in an environment of ethical principlism, with its focus on patient privacy and autonomy. Clinical genetic testing and tissue banking utilize protocols that rest on a combination of autonomy and beneficence, incorporated into codes of professional practice. Exceptions occur under a case-based rubric, but these departures are the minority. Public health, with its emphasis on the common good and general welfare of the greater population, invokes additional ethical-legal features such as the "*parens patriae*" doctrine and a spectrum of means to assure health that go beyond traditional consent. This protective legal blanket moves solidaristic and communitarian principles to the forefront. In our piece we look at significant new developments in the genomics field – family risk assessment (using family health history and cascade genetic screening) and population biobanking. We describe new forms of consent that have arisen in response to group-level genetic interventions, as well as the conflicts and compromises that arise with institutional privacy rules. The shift towards a public health ethics calls for a form of synergistic ethics in which benefits to any one individual mutually enhance benefits to all in need. This enlarged ethical perspective aims at a concept of personalized risk assessment and management in the context of public, as opposed to strictly individual, health.

Keywords: Genetics, ethics, public health policy, family health history, cascade screening, biobanks, education, legislation, professional standards, surveillance

INTRODUCTION: CURRENT TRENDS AND PAST PRECEDENTS IN GENETICS AND ETHICS

No sooner had the Human Genome Project (HGP) yielded a complete working draft of the human genome in February 2001 than scientists voiced the need to map out blocks of human genetic variation – haplotypes – dotting the genetic landscape. The new agenda was an admission that the fruits of the painstaking research would not become relevant if the population meaning of genetic discoveries was not taken into account. Further downstream, scientists envisioned employing knowledge of individual genetic variation to predict response to cancer drugs and possible toxicities that might arise. This ambition, known as "personalized medicine," would depend on the pooling of genetic information from many individuals into databases that would store collective data. No matter what phase of the genetic translational enterprise one is referring to, individual results and interventions depend on population-level knowledge. Public health, whether in the United States (the Centers for Disease Control and Prevention Office of Public Health Genomics; CDC-OPHG) or abroad (the European Centre for Public Health Genomics), has long prepared for the spillage of genetic interventions into the medical mainstream affecting large portions of the population. Policy makers are also aware that the widespread use of genetic technology carries with it public health ethical, legal, and social implications ("PHELSI") that require analysis not just at the personal but also at the population level for buy-in and appropriate application of new genetic technologies to occur [1].

Part of the dilemma in focusing on the low-hanging fruit of the HGP is that the earlier genetic discoveries, which mapped out conditions like cystic fibrosis and Duchenne muscular dystrophy, addressed single gene conditions that represent only a small portion of the genetic variations that affect health. The vast majority of human illnesses are either polygenic, involving multiple genetic loci, or multifactorial, resulting from a combination of small inherited variations in genes acting in concert with environmental factors. Examples of the former include familial breast and ovarian cancer (FBOC) and inherited cardiac arrhythmias, and of the latter diabetes, heart disease, and complex cancers. These more common but genetically complex conditions command the attention of public health practitioners. By way of contrast, clinical geneticists often find themselves in the position of utilizing genetic testing and counseling for the rarer single gene conditions requiring immediate attention.

A principlist ethical framework stressing autonomy, beneficence, non-maleficence, and justice has evolved to handle the conduct of genetic testing and counseling. The framework pays heed to the disastrous history of genetics in the first half of the twentieth century in which people placed their trust in a crude form of genetics practice – eugenics – and in forms of medical/public health investigation, such as the U.S. Public Health Service's Syphilis Study at Tuskegee, which lacked an ethical guidance structure [2]. In the United States, the 1979 Belmont Report answered such historic indiscretions with an organized set of ethical principles to underlie biomedical research [3]. As new, legitimate forms of genetic testing arose and genetic medicine struggled to divorce itself from its eugenics past, the patient's decision making capacity also gained ascendency alongside the professional's expertise, again calling for ethical principles that respected individual patients' decisions and values preferences.

Patient judgment and the personal values of health care consumers are also deeply respected by public health practitioners. The American Public Health Association (APHA) Code of Ethics for Public Health has among its principles of ethical practice respect for the rights of individuals in the community as well as respect for the diverse values, beliefs, and cultures in the community [4]. Because of its community outlook, PHELSI stresses the welfare of the collective in conjunction with the autonomy of the individual [1]. Science is used to further the health of the population, of which individuals and families are a part.

In this paper we will explore the distinctive group-oriented emphasis of public health ethics and the modalities health practitioners use to conduct their programs in an ethical manner. The interventions to be considered are a central focus of public health genetics at this very moment – use of family health histories, a form of expanded genetic screening – cascade screening among relatives, and the harnessing of population biobanks for public health ends. Certain commonalities will appear in the categories of ethical consideration belonging to these major forms of intervention. Part of the task also lies in excavating the ethical contrasts which emerge between clinical and public health practice and between these three interventional baskets. The overall intent is to build an ethical framework for a continuum of technologies. This comprehensive treatment will show that personalized medicine in the genetics arena depends on population-level activities. The application of genetic interventions to groups is not straightforward, however. Dilemmas naturally arise, which a comprehensive ethical framework can be used to address.

From Personal Autonomy to Group Benefit

Clinical medicine emphasizes the principle of autonomy in dealings with patients and research participants. A patient's approval to undergo a diagnostic or therapeutic procedure is the sine qua non of medical practice. Respect for persons is also a major pillar in biomedical research. It is carried out via an adequate informed consent, which guarantees an informed decision on the part of the research participant. Fulda and Lykens cite a case example of a 55 year-old female dialysis patient identified as a carrier of autosomal dominant polycystic kidney disease (APKD) [5]. As a result of the mother's testing, the four sons also receive genetic testing and are likewise identified as carriers. The sons' being informed of their mother's genetic status allows them each to make their own testing decision.

Genetic testing can sometimes be conducted under extenuating circumstances where patients request information that cannot be accurately known given test limitations, this information being perceived as vital to the individual's future planning. An HGP era example would be a patient's requesting their CAG repeat length from Huntington's disease genetic testing, an approximate reflection of potential longevity which became acceptable for patient disclosure only after genetic counselors gained acquaintance with the test's predictive power. Early on the issuance of repeat length was performed on a case-by-case basis, which falls under the heading of casuistric rather than principle-based ethics.

The upshot of the above APKD case was that each of the sons fully exercised their right to know their genetic status. The 30 year-old son, in order to save his wife from insurance burdens, sold their home and divorced. The 32 year-old son, father of a six year-old child, committed suicide. The case illustrates the free exercise of individual autonomy, as well as the value of pre- and posttest counseling, especially for late-onset conditions resulting in mortality. Thorough counseling might have enabled family members to exercise their right not-to-know. The condition is an intra-familial one. The mother's test results impacted her children in a major way. One sibling's handling of his own results likely tipped the balance on another's decision making. Additionally, as Fulda and Lykens point out, "... it should not be forgotten that the decision to make dialysis machines available – for example in the case of the 55 year-old mother – is a societal one" [5]. The ethical pertinence of an expansion in scope from the individual to the family and community levels is echoed in an editorial by Thomas et al. on the APHA Code of Ethics in Public Health:

> Interdependence is the complement to autonomy, a dominant principle in medical ethics. Without denying that individuals have a right to some role in decisions that affect them, a recognition of interdependence serves as a correction to an overly individualistic perspective that is inconsistent with public health's concern with whole communities and populations. [4]

The freedoms exercised pertain to the individual as well as the community so long as others are affected either by the individual's decision, as might occur in the family context, or the mode of decision making employed, which can be a societal choice. As Knoppers points out, however, thinking at the level of groups and populations requires a vetting of current ethical and legal principles towards a concept of the public good, or minimally speaking, "common" goods [6].

The idea of public goods has its roots with the 18th century philosopher David Hume, who coined the expression "providing for the 'common good'" in his *Treatise of Human Nature* [6, 7]. In Hume's definition of a "pure" public good, one person's or group's use does not preclude another's, which would seem to preserve the modern day principle of autonomy, and no one can be excluded from benefiting from a public good, which emphasizes the justice principle belonging to both biomedical and public health ethics. In contemporary times, Hannah Arendt noted, "Throughout his life man moves constantly within what is his *own* and he also moves in a sphere that is *common* to him and his fellow men" [8].

The notion of common goods also has an historic legal basis and tie to public health. In the constitutional tradition, the common good refers to individuals' welfare considered as a group, the public, or people generally. The "body politic" and "commonwealth" were the terms used in the early days of the American Republic. The commonwealth doctrine helped shape health and welfare regulatory powers in Massachusetts and throughout the United States. Each year the Massachusetts Medical Society sponsors a Shattuck Lecture on a topic of pressing medical and social significance. The lecture is named after Lemuel Shattuck, an early Massachusetts legislator and author of the 1850 Massachusetts Sanitary Commission *Report* to the state legislature. The *Report* accepted the existence of a public realm deserving of governmental protection to assure public health.

The Commonwealth, while respecting individual property rights, deserved protection for the collective good of its members. Ethical rights, if they are to be enforced, translate into policy in the form of common and statutory law. Massachusetts, with its strong Commonwealth tradition, was the first state to refer to a "police power" (*Gibbons v. Ogden*, 1824) to regulate public health: "Inspection laws, quarantine laws, health laws of every description … are component parts of this mass" [9]. Scholars interpret the case in a double sense: (1) the state has the power to constitutionally restrict private interests; and (2) the state can exercise measures to assure hygiene, seeing to it that communities live in health and safety [10].

In 1905, the United States Supreme Court, in *Jacobson v. Massachusetts*, upheld a Cambridge, Massachusetts ordinance requiring compulsory vaccination in a smallpox outbreak. While the case may be viewed as an instance of the exercise of police power, minors are often the beneficiaries of vaccination, which invokes another legal doctrine – "*parens patriae*." This doctrine refers to the state's role as sovereign and guardian of persons under legal disability, e.g., minors and incompetent persons [10].

Once again, scholars conceive of this doctrine both in the narrow sense – (1) restricting injury to others; and (2) broader sense – limiting liberty in the public realm in order to assure health, fluoridation and protection of the rights of HIV/AIDS victims being the latest examples [9, 10]. Together, these legal doctrines spell-out the province of public health – care for the health of individuals through assuring collective health. The Massachusetts Constitution defined governmental action in terms of a social compact. The whole people covenants with each citizen, and each citizen covenants with the whole people towards the common good.

THE COMMUNITARIAN CHARACTER OF PUBLIC HEALTH

A focus on the common good has prompted authors to elaborate on the distinctive features of the public health enterprise. Leo ten Kate describes clinical genetics as a field concerned with individual persons or couples or families who have or fear a health problem [11]. Public health, he states, tends to prefer a group approach to an individual one. The medical model, while it sometimes takes up the banner of primary (before-the-fact) prevention, usually sets its sights on secondary and tertiary prevention, after disease has manifested. A population approach is most feasibly carried out on the level of prevention in those at risk, before disease has manifested. Public health action tends towards the entire population and its at-risk subgroups, and ideally is anticipatory of disease. These features constitute the first two points of the Public Health Code of Ethics. The first point states: "Public health should address principally the fundamental causes of disease and requirements for health, aiming to prevent adverse health outcomes." The second point, cited earlier, regards the rights of individuals in the community. A genetics explication of the Code of Ethics acknowledges that the starting place for public health is the good of the community. The community must be well informed and public health policies should receive input from community members. But individuals must also continue to exercise their right to informed consent for genetic testing. Further, genetic testing should never be used to "create divisions between people [which] have no biological basis" [12].

The stress on community benefit can be framed by utilitarian theory – the greatest happiness of the greatest number. Indeed, utilitarian theory provides the ethical basis for mass immunization and newborn screening, as well as cost-effectiveness analyses justifying the implementation of many public health programs. Utilitarian theory does tend to clash with a number of ethical principles when a person's freedom to make the most intimate choices is compromised, and when various subgroups do not receive commensurate levels of health services [13]. Such arguments have compelled the creation of pragmatic frameworks for public health ethics where rungs of ethical importance – program goals, benefits, burdens, and fairness – are considered in step-wise fashion [14].

Authors have also suggested a refinement of the carrying out of ethical principles by creating graded options for preserving the individual's values in situations where common good is also being targeted. Chadwick and Berg, for example, have advocated the introduction of different stages of consent in sample collection for genetic databases [15].

The first step they propose is consent to entry into a sample collection, then to specific research on the samples, and finally more general research. The protocol respects autonomy, but in the background lurks a spirit of solidarity, the desire to lend mutual aid and assistance to others, often on a societal scale. They argue that in a society where one is a beneficiary of medical advancements, a person also has a duty to facilitate research progress and to provide knowledge that could be crucial to others' health:

> Family members share genes, their fates are intertwined and there are moral considerations in favour of sharing information that could benefit the whole group (one's family), even if the people providing information or samples cannot themselves benefit. [15]

Ethical principles are more situation-specific than ethical theories, which can guide the use of ethical principles, weighing and exchanging them as needed. In general, public health legal and ethical literature revolves around a communitarian language [9]. Communitarianism looks to the shared values, ideals, and goals of a community to set social policy [13]. The common good, as opposed to individual welfare, is the objective. The health of the public is one such shared value. Beauchamp and Steinbock go so far as to classify public health as a “species of communitarianism” [9]. While a utilitarian calculus may be used to decide which conditions should be tested for in newborn screening, communitarianism provides the basis for subsidy of the testing and metabolic follow-up. Society's members value the health of their youngest to the extent that they would be willing to support the health of all newborns collectively.

Communitarianism is one pole of an ethical fulcrum that also contains the other extreme of libertarianism. Libertarianism looks to individual values and goals as the arbiters of decisions. Often times it refers to an absence of governmentally-imposed restraint, though people can be guarded as to the actions of other actors, such as researchers and health care systems, as well. A tension, therefore, exists in the actions taken by public health authorities. A similar circumstance exists in the medical arena in clinical equipoise. Researchers begin a clinical trial under the assumption that no difference in efficacy exists between one trial arm and another. The null hypothesis can be dispelled as the trial proceeds, compelling ethical argument about when the trial should be stopped. Public health uses the same kind of logic in comparing interventions from observational studies. Large scale prospective studies and meta-analyses can be used to provide the decisive justification for one intervention over another. More crucially, though, in the design phase, medical and public health researchers must choose among three options – the standard approach, an alternative approach, or no intervention.

However, in research, often only two options are chosen, based on empirical reasoning and ethical choices. Even in practice, as opposed to research, public health authorities must act in a proportionate way, choosing an intervention or interventions that will improve the collective good while interfering the least with personal prerogative, achieving as much equipoise as possible [10]. The noted tension plays-out in ethical solution seeking to overcome blockades to the implementation and promotion of genetic technologies.

Public Health Ethics Applied to Three Group-Level Genetic Interventions

While genetic testing, counseling, and individualized treatment form the bread and butter of genetics in the medical mainstream, public health must concern itself with approaches that are preventive and act at the group level. "Group" here refers to families, communities, and populations. The three group-level interventions to be assessed from an ethical point of view are use of family health history (FHH), cascade screening among family members, and population biobanking. Although education is an integral part of informed consent for each of these three categories, in public health it is a modality that often stands on its own as a way to raise awareness in the community about programs being instituted.

The array of ethical concerns for public health interventions stretch from education and informed consent to stigmatization and discrimination. Table 1. lists the primary ethical considerations common to each of the three types of intervention. In keeping with recent developments, a row has also been added for the ethics of electronic means of information storage and communication.

Table 1. Ethical considerations for three public health genetics interventions

	Use of family health history	Cascade genetic screening	Population biobanking
Educational strategies	Annual Surgeon General's "My Family Health Portrait" campaign [16]	Healthy People 2020 [17], Advocacy organization awareness raising [18]	Multimedia public education campaigns [19], Public consultation [20]
Consent	3rd Party consent [21]	Direct and Indirect contact, Right Not-to-Know vs. Right-to-Know [18,22]	Broad and Blanket consent [19], Community values advisory committees [23], Public consultation [24]
Privacy & confidentiality	Controlled by family members and research team	Controlled by proband and relatives, and research team [22]	Anonymization and double-coding [19]
Stigmatization & discrimination	Attention to sensitivity of information [25]	Life insurance institutional policies [22], Health insurance - GINA	Regulatory policy for non-health-related uses [26]
Computer-based considerations	Surveillance system incorporation [27], Electronic health records policies [28]	Database use; index case identification versus relative contact [29,30]	Selective control of information use [31], Decentralized databanks and firewalls [32]

Example 1: Use of Family Health History

Family health history (FHH) is a simple yet powerful tool to assess risk for single gene diseases as well as more genetically complex common, chronic disorders in family members. Family history has come to be viewed as an independent variable in disease genesis, offering a global reflection of both genetic and environmental factors. Significant reviews have been compiled both for the effectiveness of family history [33] and its use in public health practice [34]. Williams and Hunt in the Health Family Tree Study at the University of Utah estimated FHH's cost to be about $10 per proband, making it considerably less expensive than genetic testing, and earning it the title of "first genetic test" [35]. FHH can be used to triage family members into low, medium, and high risk categories, the latter meriting referral for genetic counseling and possible genetic testing [36].

Turoldo writes about a noncoercive level of public health intervention, this category contrasting with the more concerted "soft coercive" and "highly coercive" varieties:

> Noncoercive interventions are those interventions that simply monitor the situation, that provide information, that enable individuals to change their behaviors by offering psychological or material support, or that guide choice through changing the default policy. [37]

The major public educational effort to promote the use of FHH is the Surgeon General's "My Family Health Portrait" campaign, which provides an online tool for family members to download, fill-out, and take to their healthcare provider [16]. Announcement of the Portrait and web site occurs annually around Thanksgiving; it is suggested that the holiday provides the perfect opportunity, while family members are gathered, to complete the form together. The Portrait is a good example of a dual family- and population-oriented tool to assess risk in a noncoercive way. The use of family history has also been promoted in school high schools [35], community, and church events [38] to raise health awareness and promote the taking of family history, all in a way that also maximizes individual autonomy.

It must be remembered that autonomy refers not only to the proband – to the person sent the research letter or starting the chain of family inquiry – but also to his or her relatives. Classically, the federal Common Rule 45 CFR 46.102(f) did not explicitly contemplate the extent of consent and privacy rights in "secondary" or "indirect" subjects. Awareness of the need for greater protections came about as the result of the Virginia Commonwealth University case [21]. In this case, the father of a woman being recruited for a twin study contacted federal regulators over breach of privacy. The survey instrument she had received asked questions of a private nature concerning the health behavior of family members. The federal decision was in favor of the father's position. Professional organizations such as the American Society of Human Genetics (ASHG) and the American Society of Clinical Oncology (ASCO) made adjustments in their policies concerning third parties, such as family members, after the case. The proposed revisions to the Common Rule issued in 2011 include a single informed consent process that can be applied uniformly to different types of research participants. Some criticism has been levied against the possibility of developing a single process for disparate specialized populations, which include children, groups of family members, and disaster victims [39]. Until a uniform consent policy is established, the ASHG policy, that investigators should pay close attention to the information being obtained on family members, serves as a model to other organizations.

In the non-research setting, privacy and confidentiality are controlled by: (1) those family members who assemble to fill-out a family history; and (2) the family member and health professional who together discuss the family history. Online FHH instruments keep inputed information private or within the province of the research team. In a cohort study of Health Heritage, an 89-condition web-based family history tool, 75 percent of participants said they were willing to share their risk assessment with family members, but only 39.6 percent, upon questioning, had actually done so (39.6% also responded that they were "somewhat satisfied" with the confidentiality provided by Health Heritage) [40]. Family members have a great deal of autonomy in what information they release, and sometimes do exercise their privacy. In the orbit beyond the family circle, the federal Health Insurance Portability and Accountability Act (HIPAA) governs release and exchange of family history information, just as it does the personal medical history.

Authors have commented on the type of health information that can be gathered on family members [21,25]. Information on physical conditions, such as cancer and diabetes, tends to be viewed as having less sensitivity than behavioral characteristics, such as sexual history; smoking, alcohol, and drug use; and mental health history. A family member can also be stigmatized by information that impacts their job performance (e.g., a family history of Huntington disease or heart disease in critical occupational settings). Standards of practice cover disclosure of information in situations of potential harm. Family history information containing identifiers is the property of the family itself and the family's contact(s) within the health system.

In the past, authors have dealt with security concerns for FHH information from the standpoint of conventional research studies. The "leakiness" of private telephone surveys as opposed to letter surveys, proper training of research personnel in confidentiality, and security coding are among the techniques that have been recommended to avoid breach of confidentiality [25]. The security landscape has become somewhat complicated by the existence of online risk assessment tools (e.g., Family Health*Link*, Your Disease Risk, Health Heritage in process), but these resources are university-based, and lack a commercial purpose for retaining information.

Currently FHH information is in the process of being incorporated into more massive information systems on a state and national scale. At least seven states have included questions about family history of chronic disease in their Behavioral Risk Factor Surveillance System (BRFSS) surveys. Health departments in Michigan, Minnesota, and Utah have analyzed existing clinical data on cancer family health history by accessing doctor's office chart reviews, electronic medical records, and information from local public health encounters [27]. Such data are appropriately anonymized, the ideal being for removal of identifiers at the earliest stage following collection while still allowing analysis and production of aggregate results. The U.S. Department of Health and Human Services (HHS) Personalized Health Care Initiative is also leading, via efforts of the American Health Information Community's Family Health History Multi-Stakeholder Workgroup, to the formulation of policy anticipating widespread incorporation of personal health records, including FHH, into electronic health records systems [28]. One goal is for patients, authorized family members, and their providers to receive updated pedigree and FHH information, so anonymization is out of the question. Safeguards for privacy, confidentiality, and security acceptable to all stakeholders are part of the acknowledged consensus building that needs to take place for such developments to enhance rather than detract from the common good.

Example 2: Cascade Genetic Screening

The third step in the HHS Personalized Health Care Initiative, return of newly constructed pedigree and family health history information, leads to a logical next step that these blueprints together with other information retrieved from genomic repositories will lead to the selection of genetic tests [28]. Family-based screening can often start with taking a family history of the proband and end in genetic testing of relatives [22]. Cascade genetic testing, or more properly, screening, involves communicating an individual's health information, typically their genetic test status, to their relatives so they become knowledgeable about a shared familial risk [41]. This trajectory is mirrored by the U.S. Centers for Disease Control and Prevention's Office of Public Health Genomics' vision of making cascade screening a widespread possibility [42]. The information transmission pattern resembles a snowball, where the results from an initial proband are passed to a first-degree relative. That relative's results are transmitted to another close first-or second-degree relative, who then gets tested, and so on. Those tested occupy an expanding circle of relatives – cascade screening can be quite an efficient process. Ethics enters into the decisions made since it is personal genetic information that is being transmitted from one relative to another, often in the context of a community program.

Significant progress has been made with cascade screening in Europe. In 2008 the United Kingdom's National Institute for Health and Clinical Excellence (NICE) recommended cascade screening in relatives of individuals with familial hypercholesterolemia (FH), a condition associated with premature heart attacks. Numerous articles on the practicalities and ethics of FH cascade screening have emerged from Europe [43]. Tier 1 conditions are those disease entities for which genetic testing has been strongly validated on grounds of analytical and clinical validity and utility [44]. Other Tier 1 conditions – FBOC and hereditary non-polyposis colorectal cancer (HNPCC or Lynch syndrome) – have received considerable attention from professional organizations within the United States, with recommendations in favor of cascade screening [43], yet concerted screening programs are lacking. Bowen et al. observe: "... implementation will be complex in the US because it must occur within a health care system that, unlike many European countries and Canada, is not interconnected or centrally coordinated, and in which exists widely varying coverage depending on individual insurance plans and resources" [42]. FBOC is on the list of preventive services covered under the Patient Protection and Affordable Care Act, but aside from popular recognition by Healthy People 2020 for family referral, is not being promoted as an entity for cascade genetic screening [17]. It is possible to call on disease advocacy organizations to increase awareness of the importance of screening family members for such conditions (FH has a prevalence of 1 in 500 persons in most Western countries), an approach taken in the Netherlands [18].

The informed consent process always starts with testing of a single individual, who is then asked for their permission to inform relatives [41]. When permission is granted, relatives are then either informed directly by health professionals, or indirectly through their family member [22,41]. Newson and Humphries argue that the values concerned may differ between the clinical investigation team, the proband, relatives, and broader society, which can cause tensions along ethical lines [22]. Society has an interest in reducing morbidity and mortality and thereby keeping healthcare costs down. The simple relaying of unexpected risk information, even just the index case's, may violate a relative's right not-to-know, however, and lead to psychological harm. Counters to this argument are that circumstances differ from other forms of pre-symptomatic screening lacking an effective treatment for a potentially fatal condition, and that the degree of harm caused is minimal and temporary. Additional ethical arguments for contacting relatives cited in the literature are that relatives' right-to-know about a serious, preventible condition should not be abrogated [18]; that contacting relatives in the case of Tier 1 conditions constitutes a moral duty and an ethical imperative [18,22]; and that "the patient is the family," i.e., the family members' right to informed consent in cascade screening should be respected just like the proband's [18]. The third argument shows the expansive nature of the ethical rights being considered. Simplistic as it may be, the very fact that relatives in cascade screening as opposed to the filling-out of a family history will be asked to contribute a blood sample compels contact for the purpose of informed consent.

The ethical grounding of privacy and confidentiality differs slightly for the proband versus their relatives. Historically, cascade screening programs have depended largely on indirect contact [41]. Only a small percentage of index cases decline to inform their relatives [41]. Initial family member contact by the proband allows them to judge the readiness of the relative to engage in genetic testing and receive information about his or her self, but it can also result in the proband's disclosure of their own testing status. A compromise approach respecting the proband's right to privacy, which also increases the relative's decisional autonomy, is for them to be provided a general leaflet for distribution to family members prior to further contact [22]. Several countries – the United States, France, Greece, and Denmark – have adopted policies that prohibit or do not support direct contact by investigators [41].

Information diffusion within the family can be more nuanced than expected. A qualitative study of family communication about HNPCC genetic testing revealed proband readiness to share news of a genetic mutation with spouse, children, and siblings, but reluctance to do so with nieces, nephews, and cousins [45]. Direct contact of relatives by the professional team can help by maximizing privacy of the proband's genetic information. From a public health standpoint, it also maximizes the chances of being able to contact additional at-risk relatives, a methodology that has been likened to contact tracing [22]. Direct contact by the investigative team is, therefore, the preferred method in the United Kingdom and the Netherlands [41]. Relatives, however, may be less willing to share news of a mutation than the proband. A compromise procedure has been suggested for direct contact whereby relatives' names and addresses are not *recorded* in the cascade screening register until they have themselves consented [22].

It could be argued that communication of genetic risk status between family members, either before or after direct contact, carries with it the potential for stigma. Unlike the stigmatization noted in premarital genetic testing, though, all family members are at risk. In cascade screening the family is an integral unit. Regarding societal discrimination, in many countries life insurance premiums for life expectancy curtailing conditions such as FH can be raised or lowered depending on whether the condition is well-treated [22]. The ethics of life insurance are different from the ethics of health insurance, with actuarial fairness playing a much larger role in the former, and communitarian concerns having a more prominent place in the latter. It is important that countries have health insurance-related legislative protections for genetic testing in place, analogous to the Genetic Information Nondiscrimination Act (GINA) in the United States, before major population screening is implemented.

O'Kane et al. have argued that an effective, large-scale cascade screening program cannot be undertaken without a suitable database to allow full documentation of family trees, screening status, and screening results in family members [46]. Checks have been made on the feasibility of electronically identifying index cases of Tier 1 conditions from primary care clinical records. Gray et al. identified 12 definite and 8 probable cases of FH from computer and notes searches of 402 patients in a South London practice, 9 of whom were not previously known to have FH [29]. However, one study of computerized Duchenne muscular dystrophy registry use and letter send-out in West of Scotland and South East Thames, United Kingdom failed to demonstrate increased levels of carrier testing compared to more informal, non-computer-based registries [30]. Cascade screening in the community setting is only as effective as the means used to contact at-risk family members.

Example 3: Population Biobanking

At a certain size threshold, health information needs to be stored in a centralized repository making it more manageable and accessible. Hospitals have a longstanding history of storing pathology samples in paraffin blocks, accessing them when the derived information will be helpful for patient treatment and related disease research. Population biobanks expand the concept to a population-wide level. On the international front, population biobanks now exist in myriad countries, including the United Kingdom, Iceland, Canada, Sweden, Estonia, Japan, Latvia, and Singapore. The United States Department of Health and Human Services has undertaken activities evaluating the possibility of a large-scale (1 million person strong) cohort study of genes, environment, and disease, a project which is yet to occur. Nevertheless, major healthcare systems in the United States – the Mayo Health Clinic in Minnesota, Marshfield Clinic in Wisconsin, Kaiser Permanente in

California, and Veterans Health Administration in Washington, D.C. – have established biobanks that mirror on a regional level what has transpired nationally in other countries. While these efforts have many applications in pharmacogenomics and personalized medicine, health departments in a number of states, Michigan, Connecticut, and California, have either planned or established repositories that can be used for public health purposes. Denmark as well has a newborn screening register and biobank. These biobanks require special ethical attention because their continuity rests on individual willingness and public need, two forces that do not always intersect.

Of all the interventions discussed in this paper, biobanks depend the most on an atmosphere of transparency and an effort at public education. The Icelandic Biobank partnering with deCODE Genetics was preceded by a public campaign involving 700 newspaper articles, more than 100 radio and television programs, and several town hall meetings spread across Iceland [19]. The UK Biobank hosted 8 consultations with various public groups before it was established [20]. A web site was constructed listing the results of public and stakeholder consultations, committee members' names and biographies, and reviewers' reports on scientific protocol. Lay members were also on the committee developing the ethics and governance framework. The consequences of ignoring the public are dire. The Tongan Biobank was abandoned after awarding an exclusive licensing agreement between the Tongan government and a private biotechnology company without a public forum for discussion. Numerous advocacy groups expressed vehement criticism of the project [19]. In Minnesota, lack of public understanding of the utility and ethical use of newborn dried blood spots prompted a statewide campaign against their use by the Citizen's Council for Health Freedom. In Texas, a federal law suit prompted the Department of State Health Services to destroy ~4.5 million stored blood spots [24]. These two sets of examples show the immense value of public education and consultation, which ultimately address ethical issues, such as parental consent and sharing of benefits, of great interest to the public.

Because of the vast number of participants involved, biobanks are most appropriately couched in several layers of consent. Methodologies such as community review and community consultation have been used with community-based research. Consultation in the form of public forums, town hall meetings, and focus groups is of value because it allows public input before biobank design is completed and during the early stages of operation [23,24]. Inclusion in biobank ethics or community values advisory committees represents a second level of active, vocal participation, one that extends through time [23]. Ideally the participation involves lay inclusion on the committee or board itself. Individual consent is the third level of autonomy. Consent must take into account policy for samples and records existing prior to and after establishment of the biobank. For the Michigan Neonatal Biobank, the Michigan Department of Community Health Institutional Review Board (IRB) granted a waiver of consent for the 4 million dried blood spots that had been stored before May 1, 2010 [23]. Opt-out is available for persons who do not want their pre-2010 blood spots to be available for research, but community meetings have suggested that many residents are unaware of the very existence of the Biobank [24]. Parent or legal guardian signed consent is required for research on newborn blood spots taken after the May 2010 date. Sensitivity is required in this state-run biobank and others to achieve consents that are genuinely informed. Secondary use of samples beyond the originally stated use creates a standing dilemma for many varieties of biobank, with solutions varying from opt-out for particular uses, to broad consent, to blanket consent for all purposes [19]. Public health biobanks generally operate under blanket consent since they are not created to address just one genre of research, yet the research areas they do address must apply to the standard of serving the public good. Those charged with oversight must not assume that the public nature of state-run biobanks removes the need for public education about them.

Three main methods are used to protect the confidentiality of biobank donors: (1) full anonymization of samples and removal of identifiers from the start; (2) initial anonymization of samples with removal of identifiers after accomplishment of the originally intended use; and (3) double-coding, involving maintenance of a secure code linking samples given project identification numbers with personally identifying information [19]. The ethical equation is more complicated with public health biobanks which are built around biological samples, e.g., newborn dried blood spots, which may have immediate or more remote preventive purposes involving familial disease.

The concept of confidentiality is eroded from two different quarters by genetic biobanks. First, maverick research has shown that it is easier than expected to re-identify persons participating in public sequencing and personalized genomics projects [47]. Research organizations are moving in the direction of establishing professional sanctions for such occurrences [48]. Sanction mechanisms are already in place in the United Kingdom in case any violation of UK Biobank confidentiality policies occurs. Secondly, should possibly beneficial discoveries be made, the participating public may not want total removal of identifiers [19]. Corresponding input during public consultation caused the Canadian CARTaGENE project to shift its policy from anonymization of samples to double-coding. This approach also has advantages for longitudinal research in which participant medical or health information is periodically updated [49].

For the most part, findings generated by biobanks are reported in aggregate form, making it very difficult to use them for discriminatory purposes. GINA was passed to outlaw genetic discrimination on the part of health insurers and employers. Biobank participants may still have concerns about untoward uses of their samples or personal health information. For example, in a paternity suit in 1999, the High Court in New Zealand was asked for release of a recently deceased child's blood sample for DNA analysis, which it granted [26]. Several forensic uses of biobank tissue samples exist which people would view as intrusive. These uses are not health-related. Kharaboyan et al. suggest, "Introducing regulatory policies and security measures to regulate the length of sample retention and access to identifiable samples will help insure that [dried blood spots] do not automatically end up as part of law enforcement or government DNA databases, or in the hands of other third parties ..." [26]. Although in the past electronic systems provoked fears of loss of privacy and violation of security, in the present they are providing solutions to several of the above ethical dilemmas. For distributed samples and data from different biobanks, cohort or associational studies that are being combined, methods have been developed to pool and analyze the *calculations* from harmonized individual-level data at the various centers, rather than the individualized data itself [32]. This approach keeps individual data behind multi-center firewalls, inaccessible to outside parties. Other systems allow biobank contributors to selectively prespecify what type of personal identifying or health information they want to make available downstream, and for what types of research organizations and health researchers [31]. Electronic systems can be used not only for informational purposes but to assure ethical use of the information as well.

Summary of Common Themes Along a Population Trajectory

The interventions described move markedly beyond a strictly individualistic orientation, and of necessity arc back to public health ethics. In the clinical setting information provision and explanations offered by the healthcare provider are sufficient openers before an examination. In the three examples given, some degree of public education is needed as well. Family health history offers an example of education rallying around a unifying national campaign; population biobanking an example of multiple campaigns, one tailored for each biobank. The consequences of foregoing public transparency and education are dire when society is the program participant.

The consent process billows out over the three categories of intervention like an unfolding umbrella. The filling-out of FHH always starts out with one willing person, though family members can end-up helping. Consent in cascade screening is offered by each family member contacted. Autonomy in population biobanking is exercised at three levels – two group-oriented, and one individual. Confidentiality in the use of FHH and cascade screening is between the index person and their family members, with responsibility for ethical handling of familial information on the part of the provider. With biobanks larger policy formulations – professional regulations and legislation – are needed. The leakiness of information is spread across society.

The greater concern with stigmatization from inadvertant disclosure of FHH information is occupational, whereas with cascade screening, since it relies on system-level coordination, it is insurance-related. The more than ten years it took to pass GINA were well worth it given the volume of genetic testing and data collection that can occur with cascade screening and population biobanking. Biobank information, like that obtained by direct-to-consumer genetic testing companies, would seem to perfectly fit with many non-health-related uses, which is exactly why it is in need of cross-the-board policies – professional, legal, and regulatory – that would restrict its use to constructive health purposes. Nondiscrimination policies for all three categories of intervention go beyond the province of traditional medical institutions.

When Georgetown University's Laurence Gostin wrote of an emergent "health information infrastructure" in 1996, it was a multi-tentacled beast that connected one's healthcare records with workplace screens and criminal justice records, a very dangerous creature, indeed [50]. In a sign of progress, the electronic face of this infrastructure is allowing family history information to find population relevance in public health surveillance systems and electronic health records systems. It is actually offering a solution to several ethical dilemmas that face biobanks, a result of the biobank ideal to help everyone without harming anyone.

Ethical Concerns Distinctive to Public Health

While Thomas et al. contend that interdependence is the complement to autonomy, Turoldo takes the position that "responsibility" occupies this spot [37]. The two perspectives do not necessarily contradict each other since one is centered on ethics from a relational standpoint; the other from a view of the agents involved. It has been stated that public health, because it employs coercive measures for the good of others and the whole, continues to be paternalistic. Medicine has been shifting away from paternalism. In actuality the types of paternalistic influence exerted by public health programs can be noncoercive – educational campaigns; softly coercive – legislation; and highly coercive – compulsory programs and population or group monitoring [37]. Much of the national legislation mentioned in this paper, such as HIPAA and GINA, affects both medical and public health activities. On the state level, public health departments have been involved with legislation that prohibits the use of genetic information in Medicare-related services, enforces access to and reporting of cancer and birth defects case information to disease registries, and enacts and molds newborn screening programs.

The paternalism being engaged in is not the usual sort because compulsion is not being levied on the patient. Assisting the patient with their decisions is the duty of the doctor or genetic counselor. Rather, as demonstrated in the three interventions covered, public health is acting on their significant others. Expanding the circle of preventive influence is the goal of family health histories and cascade screening. The ultimate outcome of biobanks is that all will benefit, even those not immediately contributing to them. Looking more closely at exactly what FHH, cascade screening, and biobanks are used for, the aim is prevention of future disease that has not yet manifested. Turoldo contrasts public health responsibility with the after-the-fact imputability for actions that have already taken place, typical of civil and penal law.

Public health is very much concerned with health for all. Point 4. of the Code of Ethics for Public Health states: "Public health should advocate for, or work for the empowerment of, disenfranchised community members, ensuring that the basic resources and conditions necessary for health are accessible to all people in the community" [12]. The egalitarian spirit is precisely why members of the public health community have engaged with members of diverse racial-ethnic groups in community dialogues to sound out their hopes and concerns with genetic technologies, and to avoid policies that only favor the health of the majority [51]. It is also why members of the academic and practicing public health communities are so eager to ensure that the Patient

Protection and Affordable Care Act's covered services impact as many groups as possible. Work is yet to be done to make sure the services are "ethically" covered. Different family members of extended families typically have different levels of healthcare coverage. BRCA1/2 breast and ovarian cancer genetic testing should be available to the array of family members; cascade screening should be covered and use of FHH should be more than a suggestion.

The flip-side of fair allocation is unfair attention to particular groups, thus resulting in discrimination. Stigmatization and discrimination are critical ethical components to any measuring up of genetic technologies. Successful dialoguing on community concerns over population-wide interventions, such as biobanking, will assess for discrimination concerns and suggestions right alongside standard ethical issues such as consent [24].

CONCLUSION: A POPULATION-BASED PERSONALIZED ETHOS

Technical and ethical comparisons of genetic technologies often follow a life course progression – from carrier and prenatal screening to newborn screening to adult predictive and diagnostic genetic testing. All of these modalities stay within the skin of the individual. The earliest public health collaboration was built around between-person disease transmission, though. In this conception, risk is spread across and moves through multiple parties, even the whole population or parts of the population. The requisite ethics is necessarily distinct from a single-person ethics.

Shared territory exists between medicine and public health when it comes to the three interventions discussed. The areas of expertise point in different directions, though. A Mayo or Marshfield Clinic will use its biobank to discover new genetic variants for more effectively treating the individual patient. Traditional autonomy, confidentiality, and beneficence are operative in this realm. A public health biobank, containing cord blood or newborn blood spots, will be used for research that will touch the larger population. Genetic variants and gene-environment interactions discovered can be used for screening which draws from and helps large numbers of people in a preventive fashion. The ethics will focus more on solidarity, sharing, and the common good. Societal benefit is the end; multiparty ethical criteria are the means.

When discussing the good of a certain intervention to society, the philosophy being employed is an "ethos," a collective framework and a new outlook. The difference between "PHELSI" and "ELSI" is more than one letter deep. The vector of attention points outwards rather than inwards. When people attend to one another from a communitarian stance, they consider a synergy of action and not just protection of the self's rights. Think how such an attitude would change the world of disease detection, information collection, and health information utilization. Genetic interventions such as personalized risk assessment would be applied to individuals, but the data underlying the interventions would derive from a maximum number of willing contributors, and the policies employed would enable many people to participate and benefit, often at the same time. Population-based knowledge, when sharing is the goal, yields the most precise and just personalized medicine.

REFERENCES

[1] Citrin T, Modell SM. Genomics and public health: ethical, legal and social issues. In: Centers for Disease Control and Prevention, Office of Genomics and Disease Prevention. Genomics and Population Health: United States, 2003. Atlanta, GA; 2004. www.cdc.gov/genomics/about/reports/2003.

[2] Tuskegee Syphilis Study Legacy Committee. Final report of the Tuskegee Syphilis Study Legacy Committee. Tuskegee, AL: Tuskegee University; 1997. exhibits.hsl.virginia.edu/badblood/report.

[3] National Commission for the Protection of Human Subjects of Biomedical and Behavioral Research. The Belmont Report: ethical principles and guidelines for the protection of human subjects of research. Washington, D.C.: U.S. Government Printing Office, DHEW Publication No. (OS) 78-0012; 1978.

[4] Thomas JC, Sage M, Dillenberg J, Guillory VJ. A code of ethics for public health. *Am J Public Health* 2002; 92(7): 1057-1060.

[5] Fulda KG, Lykens K. Ethical issues in predictive genetic testing: a public health perspective. *J Med Ethics* 2006; 32(3): 143-147.

[6] Knoppers BM. Of genomics and public health: building public "goods"? *Canadian Med Assoc J* 2005; 173(10): 1185-1186.

[7] Hume D. *A treatise of human nature*. 2nd ed. Eds. Selby-Bigge, LA, Nidditch, PH. Oxford, UK: Oxford University Press; 1739; 1978.

[8] Arendt H. *The human condition.* 2nd ed. Chicago: University of Chicago Press; 1958; 1998.

[9] Beauchamp DE. Community: the neglected tradition of public health. In: Beauchamp D, Steinbock B, eds. *New ethics for the public's health*, pp. 57-67. New York: Oxford University Press; 1999.

[10] Gostin LO. *Public health law: power, duty, restraint.* Berkeley, CA: University of California Press; 2000.

[11] Ten Kate LP. Community genetics: a bridge between clinical genetics and public health. *Community Genet* 2005; 8(1): 7-11.

[12] Thomas JC, Irwin DE, Zulker ES, Millikan RC. Genomics and the public health code of ethics. *Am J Public Health* 2005; 95(12): 2139-2143.

[13] Beauchamp D, Steinbock B. Introduction: ethical theory and public health. In: Beauchamp D, Steinbock B, eds. *New ethics for the public's health*, pp. 3-24. New York: Oxford University Press; 1999.

[14] Kass NE. An ethics framework for public health. *Am J Public Health* 2001; 91(11): 1776-1782.

[15] Chadwick R, Berg K. Solidarity and equity: new ethical frameworks for genetic databases. *Nat Rev Genet* 2001; 2(4): 318-321.

[16] Office of the Surgeon General. My Family Health Portrait. Rockville, MD: U.S. Department of Health & Human Services; 2014. https://familyhistory.hhs.gov/fhh-web/home.action.

[17] Healthy People 2020. Genomics. Washington, D.C.: U.S. Department of Health and Human Services; 2014. http://www.healthypeople.gov/2020/topicsobjectives2020/overview.aspx?topicid=15.

[18] De Wert G. Cascade screening: whose information is it anyway? *Euro J Hum Genet* 2005; 13(4): 397-398.

[19] Swede H, Stone CL, Norwood AR. National population-based biobanks for genetic research. *Genet Med* 2007; 9(3): 141-149.

[20] Levitt M. UK Biobank: a model for public engagement? *Genomics, Society and Policy* 2005; 1(3): 78-81.

[21] Botkin JR. Protecting the privacy of family members in survey and pedigree research. *J Am Med Assoc* 2001; 285(2): 207-211.

[22] Newson AJ, Humphries SE. Cascade screening in familial hypercholesterolaemia: how should family members be contacted? Euro *J Hum Genet* 2005; 13(4): 401-408.

[23] Chrysler D, McGee H, Bach J, Goldman E, Jacobson PD. The Michigan BioTrust for Health: using dried bloodspots for research to benefit the

community while respecting the individual. *J Law Med Ethics* 2001; 39 Suppl 1: 98-101.

[24] Thiel DB, Platt T, Platt J, King SB, Kardia SLR. Community perspectives on public health biobanking: an analysis of community meetings on the Michigan BioTrust for Health. *J Community Genet* 2014; 5(2): 125-138.

[25] Kendler KS. Family history information in biomedical research. *J Continuing Educ Health Professions* 2001; 12(4): 215-223.

[26] Kharaboyan L, Avard D, Knoppers BM. Storing newborn blood spots: modern controversies. *J Law Med Ethics* 2004; 32(4): 741-748.

[27] Association of State and Territorial Health Officials (ASTHO). The 2010 state public health genomics resource guide. Arlington, VA; 2010. ASTHO. http://www.astho.org/Programs/Access/Genomics/The-2010-State-Public-Health-Genomics-Resource-Guide.

[28] Feero WG, Bigley MB, Brinner KM, and the Family Health History Multi-Stakeholder Workgroup of the American Health Information Community. New standards and enhanced utility for family health history information in the electronic health record: an update from the American Health Information Community's Family Health History Multi-Stakeholder Workgroup. *J Am Med Inform Assoc* 2008; 15(6): 723-728.

[29] Gray J, Jaiyeola A, Whiting M, Modell M, Wierzbicki AS. Identifying patients with familial hypercholesterolaemia in primary care: an informatics-based approach in one primary care centre. *Heart* 2008; 94(6): 754-758.

[30] McGowan R, Challoner BR, Holloway RS, Joss S, Wilcox D, Holden ST, Tolmie J, Longman C. Results of Duchenne muscular dystrophy family screening in practice: leaks rather than cascades? *Clin Genet* 2013; 83(2): 187-190.

[31] Shelton R. Private Access, Inc. In: Genetic Alliance / Presidential Commission for the Study of Bioethical Issues. Technology – is a deeper dive needed? Washington, D.C.: Genetic Alliance; 8 Oct 2013. http://www.geneticalliance.org/sites/default/files/webinararchive/100813 Shelton.pdf.

[32] Wallace SE, Gaye A, Shoush O, Burton PR. Protecting personal data in epidemiological research: DataSHIELD and UK law. *Public Health Genomics* 2014; 17(3): 149-157.

[33] Berg AO, Baird MA, Botkin JR, Driscoll DA, Fishman PA, Guarino PD, Hiatt RA, Jarvik GP, Millon-Underwood S, Morgan TM, Mulvihill JJ,

Pollin TI, Schimmel SR, Stefanek ME, Vollmer WM, Williams JK. Natioal Institutes of Health state-of-the-science conference statement: family history and improving health. *Ann Intern Med* 2009; 151(12): 872-877.

[34] Valdez R, Yoon PW, Qureshi N, Green RF, Khoury MJ. Family history in public health practice: a genomic tool for disease prevention and health promotion. *Annu Rev Public Health* 2010; 31: 69-87.

[35] Williams RR, Hunt SC, Barlow GK, Chamberlain RM, Weinberg AD, Cooper HP, Carbonari JP, Gotto AM, Jr. Health family trees: a tool for finding and helping young family members of coronary and cancer prone pedigrees in Texas and Utah. *Am J Public Health* 1988; 78(10): 1283-1286.

[36] Yoon PW, Scheuner MT, Peterson-Oehlke KL, Gwinn M, Faucett A, Khoury MJ. Can family history be used as a tool for public health and preventive medicine? *Genet Med* 2002; 4(4): 304-310.

[37] Turoldo F. Responsibility as an ethical framework for public health interventions. *Am J Public Health* 2009; 99(7): 1197-1202.

[38] Theisen V, Duquette D, Kardia S, Wang C, Beene-Harris R, Bach J. Blood Pressure Sunday: introducing genomics to the community through family history. *Prev Chronic Disease* 2005; 2(2): A23.

[39] National Research Council, Committee on Revisions to the Common Rule for the Protection of Human Subjects in Research in the Behavioral and Social Sciences. Proposed revisions to the common rule – perspectives of social and behavioral scientists: workshop summary. Rep. Pool R. Washington, D.C.: The National Academies Press; 2013.

[40] Cohn WF, Ropka ME, Pelletier SL, Barrett JR, Kinzie MB, Harrison MB, Liu Z, Miesfeldt F, Tucker AL, Worrall BB, Gibson J, Mullins IM, Elward KS, Franko J, Guterbock TM, Knaus WA. Health Heritage © a web-based tool for the collection and assessment of family health history: initial user experience and analytic validity. *Public Health Genomics* 2010; 13(7-8): 477-491.

[41] Maxwell SJ, Molster CM, Poke SJ, O'Leary P. Communicating familial hypercholesterolemia genetic information within families. *Genet Test Molec Biomarkers* 2009; 13(3): 301-306.

[42] Bowen MS, Kolor K, Dotson WD, Ned RM, Khoury MJ. Public health action in genomics is now needed beyond newborn screening. *Public Health Genomics* 2012; 15(6): 327-334.

[43] Centers for Disease Control and Prevention – Office of Public Health Genomics (CDC-OPHG). Genomic Tests and family history by levels of

evidence. Atlanta, GA: CDC; 2014. http://www.cdc.gov/genomics/gtesting/tier.htm.

[44] Khoury MJ, Coates RJ, Evans JP. Evidence-based classification of recommendations on use of genomic tests in clinical practice: dealing with insufficient evidence. *Genet Med* 2010; 12(11): 680-683.

[45] Peterson SK, Watts BG, Koehly LM, Vernon SW, Baile WF, Kohlmann WK, Gritz ER. How families communicate about HNPCC genetic testing: findings from a qualitative study. *Am J Med Genet* 2003; 119C(1): 78-86.

[46] O'Kane MJ, Menown IB, Graham I, Maher V, Tomkin G, Nicholls P, Graham C. The detection of heterozygous familial hypercholesterolemia in Ireland. *Adv Ther* 2012; 29(5): 456-463.

[47] Vence T. Funders fight re-identication. *The Scientist*, 25 Mar 2014. http://www.the-scientist.com/?articles.view/articleNo/39544/title/Funders-Fight-Re-Identification.

[48] Ryan C. Research funders outline steps to prevent re-identification of anonymized study participants. Britain: The Wellcome Trust; 24 Mar 2014. http://www.wellcome.ac.uk/News/Media-office/Press-releases/2014/WTP055974.htm.

[49] Austin MA, Harding SE, McElroy CE. Monitoring ethical, legal, and social issues in developing population genetic databases. *Genet Med* 2003; 5(6): 451-457.

[50] Gostin LO, Lazzarini Z, Nezlund VS, Osterholm MT. The public health information infrastructure. A national review of the law on health information privacy. *J Am Med Assoc* 1996; 275(24): 1921-1927.

[51] Bonham VL, Citrin T, Modell SM, Frankli TH, Bleicher EWB, Fleck LM. Community-based dialogue: engaging communities of color in the United States' genetics policy conversation. *J Health Politics Policy Law* 2009; 34(3): 325-359.

In: Patient Rights
Editor: Jenna Pope
ISBN: 978-1-63482-136-0

Chapter 2

An Ethical Framework for the Routine Randomization of Medical Therapies

Ahmed Elsayyad*
Public Health Studies, Johns Hopkins University,
Baltimore, MD, US

Abstract

In the past 50 years, ethical concerns concerning human experimentation have arisen with the advancement of new medical research and technology. While the benefits of human experimentation are well known in the fields of biology, psychology, sociology, and medicine, the conditions of human subject research have been persistently controversial. Our current healthcare model operates based on a distinction between clinical care and clinical research. Subsequently, several bioethicists have argued that this segregated model poses several conceptual, moral and empirical problems. As a result, some have suggested blurring the line between clinical research and clinical care. One such plan to blur this line is by randomizing the type of therapy given to patients and collecting data from it if the treatment options have similar risk profiles. A potential problem with any new change in a system that monitors human subject research is the over- or under-

* Corresponding author: Ahmed Elsayyad. Public Health Studies, Johns Hopkins University, 3505 N. Charles Street, Baltimore, Maryland, US. E-mail: aelsayy1@jhu.edu.

protection of research subjects (patients in this case). In my commentary, I will highlight four potential issues that I can foresee happening under the proposal of routinely randomizing medical interventions: [i] patients' health and well-being may be compromised, [ii] patients' preferences may not be respected, [iii] patients' privacy may be violated, and [iv] physicians' judgment may be restricted. To prevent these four problems, I propose that we fulfill four criteria that are aimed to prevent the over- or under-protection of research subjects under a randomization proposal.

I. INTRODUCTION

In this chapter, I will first provide background on comparative effectiveness research (CER) and on the current movements (i.e., learning healthcare systems) in advancing such research. Second, I will describe the implementation, legal, and ethical challenges facing the advancement of CER. Third, I will identify three consent models, with two being alternatives to what we have today. Fourth, I will summarize a few empirical studies on patient opinions concerning the different consent models. Fifth, I will delineate a current proposal for an opt-out consent model for pragmatic randomized controlled trials. Sixth, I will argue for four ethical criteria that we should follow if we implemented such a proposal. Seventh, I will address the need to determine patients' opinions for randomized trials.

II. BACKGROUND

Comparative Effectiveness Research

In many contexts, we resort to the systematic evaluation of products and services to help guide our decision-making. Millions of Americans subscribe to *Consumer Reports*, a magazine that regularly reviews and compares consumer products and services, to find the product or service that best matches their needs. An evaluation by *Consumer Reports* will assess various characteristics of a product or service, such as cost, quality, and durability (Consumer Reports, 2014). Furthermore, high school seniors and parents may use a tool such as *US News and World Report College Compass* to guide them in choosing a college based on factors of ranking, academic life, campus safety, costs, and financial aid. The field of medicine lacks a comprehensive guide because very few research studies have investigated whether a particular drug works better than another drug (Green, 2006).

For many medical problems, we do not know the best way to treat patients because of the lack of research studies that compare similar interventions (Faden, 2013). This type of research that evaluates the impact of different options that are available for treating a given medical condition for a set of patients is known as comparative effectiveness research (CER) (DeMaria, 2009). CER seeks to identify the relative benefits and harms of interventions in a real-world setting (Faden, 2013). It is important to note the distinction between *efficacy* research and *effectiveness* research. Efficacy research studies investigate whether a treatment produces the desired outcome in a controlled environment (Laken, 2013). In contrast, effectiveness research studies are conducted in the real world in clinical practices, and they are intended to investigate which interventions are the most effective (Laken, 2013).

An efficacy study, for example, may investigate whether drug A treats hypertension. An effectiveness study instead will investigate whether drug A or drug B is better at treating hypertension. While it is important to conduct both efficacy and effectiveness research, most medical research today is of the former type and seeks to determine whether medicines work in the first place (Faden, 2013).

Movement to a Learning Health Care System

There have been recent proposals to develop a healthcare system that promotes comparative effectiveness research (Olsen, 2007). These proposals revolve around the idea of obtaining and analyzing electronic health records (EHR) obtained from a clinical setting to provide data for CER studies. For example, researchers have described the great need for EHR in evidence development for cancer clinical care and research (Miriovsky, 2012). They argue that, to fully utilize the potential of EHR, we should capture clinical informatics to provide mechanisms in which EHRs can facilitate comparative effectiveness research (CER). Ideally, real-time analytics of EHR data can provide improved point-of-care evidence to oncologists (Miriovsky, 2012). A practical implication of this improved point-of-care evidence could be that an oncologist could enter information about a patient with prostate cancer and receive a list of recommendations based on the current empirical evidence from all prostate cancer patients with similar characteristics.

An initiative to promote this integration of information generated by EHRs for analysis in CER studies was galvanized after the Institute of Medicine roundtable on Evidence-Based Medicine Learning Health Care System workshop in July 2006 (Olsen, 2007). This roundtable discussion convened to discuss issues of healthcare delivery so that evidence is available when needed and applied in healthcare more effectively than it is today (Olsen, 2007). Additionally, this workshop called for a reevaluation of how health care is structured to develop and apply evidence. It described the need for a “sustainable system that gets the right care to people when they need it and then captures the results of improvement. [This nation] needs a healthcare system that learns” (Olsen, 2007).

After the workshop, research around this idea of a *learning healthcare system (LHCS)*, or a model in which data generated by routine clinical care feed databases that support clinical decision support, gained momentum (Miriovsky, 2012). An LHCS is a healthcare system that both provides care to patients and routinely conducts constant research to improve the quality of care. Every time that a patient goes to a doctor, clinic, or hospital becomes an opportunity to learn and conduct research using information that doctors record about each patient. The system learns about what works and what does not work from each patient visit and changes care accordingly. This allows for the rapid accumulation of clinical information in an accessible form (Miriovsky, 2012).

Several healthcare institutions have already adopted systems that integrate electronic health information to better conduct research. I will describe three such programs of varying degrees that are already in place: the first uses electronic health records to improve recruitment for research, the second uses such health records to generate research findings, and the third uses electronic health information to provide empirical conclusions that are rapidly integrated to promote clinical care (a full learning healthcare system). First, in 2005, the US National Institutes of Health (NIH) funded the electronic Primary Care Research Network (ePCRN) as one of 12 pilot programs intended to facilitate clinical research by using primary care electronic health records (Peterson, 2006). ePRCN works to assist primary care practitioners in identifying suitable participants for research by extracting health record information (Peterson, 2006). For example, a primary care provider would be notified when a patient that he or she is treating is eligible (based on characteristics present in the health care records) to perform a research study.

The provider could then ask the patient whether the patient is interested. This is designed to make recruitment of these patients easier by extracting health care information from the patients (Delaney, 2012). Second, the Cleveland Clinic investigated the risk of coronary artery disease, congestive heart failure, and mortality using patients from their own electronic health records (Pantalone, 2009). They utilized electronic health records with CER to examine whether there was a relationship between the risk for coronary artery disease and the use of various oral diabetes medications.

Furthermore, they studied the mortality risks associated with those taking different oral diabetes medications (Pantalone, 2009). This information would be impractical to gather in a clinical trial because of the amount of time required from the point of intervention (oral diabetes medication) to the outcome (death). Consequently, this sheds light on the potential information that can be gathered by combining electronic medical records and CER in a clinical setting. Third, Kaiser Permanente integrated its health information technology and electronic health records into a large database engine that works to inform oncologists (Miriovsky, 2012).

Utilizing their electronic health records system, Kaiser has implemented several point-of-care evidence-based systems. For example, oncologists will be alerted about potential prevention options (e.g., breast cancer screening) and questionable results in x-rays and blood tests (Wallace, 2007).

Additionally, the electronic medical system can inform clinicians of standardized treatment plans for cancer patients based on evidence from patients with similar characteristics (Wallace, 2007).

As mentioned above, current healthcare systems have integrated electronic medical records to conduct comparative effectiveness research.

This integration can be used to recruit more patients from CER, to generate research, and to create a learning health care system.

III. Challenges in Integrating Electronic Medical Information and CER

While there are clear benefits to integrating electronic medical records with comparative effectiveness research, there are several limitations. There are implementation, legal, and ethical challenges that prevent the research integration of electronic medical information with comparative effectiveness research.

Implementation Challenges

There are several technical challenges that must be overcome to integrate properly the information that we obtain from electronic medical records with comparative effectiveness research. The main challenges are the lack of (1) interoperability among different electronic medical record systems, (2) standardization of electronic health records codes, (3) development of real-time analytics, and (4) access to data (Miriovsky, 2012). The first issue is that we must improve the interoperability, or the ability for a system to exchange data across sectors, of current electronic medical records systems (Miriovsky, 2012). For example, we must ensure that the information gathered from the clinical laboratory department is easily accessible to the radiology department. This makes it easier for radiologists to look at their patients' lab results. The more interoperability of electronic information is achieved, the faster the healthcare system can learn. Making electronic medical systems from different hospitals interoperable will increase the amount of patient data collected. This will increase the patient sample size used for research and ultimately increase the scientific validity of such research.

The second challenge is to increase the standardization of health record codes. The idea is that, if one health system uses the labels of "white" and "black" for race and another uses "Caucasian" and "African American," then extra variables are created that cause problems in data analysis (Miriovsky, 2012). We should create standardized codes across health care systems to improve the first challenge of interoperability and facilitate the correct analysis of data sets. The third challenge is that we must develop analytical processing systems that continuously assess the aggregating data.

To obtain a learning healthcare system that gathers new information every time a new patient is entered into the system, we must develop and incorporate an analytical processing system into the health care system. The development of such a system could begin with an initial analysis of the current electronic medical records. Then outcomes would be tracked by the system, and confidence in the evidence would grow as more patients are enrolled. This would improve the clinical support, and over time, the cycle time for analysis would decrease, which would "ultimately [reach] a state with continuous data aggregation and analysis" (Miriovsky, 2012).

The fourth challenge is to improve access to data. Even if healthcare systems were very interoperable, their data were standardized, and analytical processing systems were in place, the benefits would not be realized if there were no access to the information.

Because of legal and ethical concerns, there is an enormous challenge in accessing patient information. Without the ability to access this information, the benefits of integrating electronic medical information and comparative effectiveness research cannot be realized.

Legal Challenges

To address the fourth challenge in integrating electronic medical records and comparative effectiveness research, we must understand the legal and policy barriers to accessing electronic medical information. There are three main concerns about utilizing electronic health record data for purposes beyond treatment: (i) the variable interpretation of federal laws governing secondary uses of EHR, (ii) challenges related to IRB review, and (iii) the potential variability in state laws (McGraw, 2012).

The two most important federal laws that are related to the use of health information are the Health Insurance Portability and Accountability Act (HIPAA) and the Common Rule (McGraw, 2012). In the US, the HIPAA Privacy Rule prevents researchers from accessing practice data to identify subjects for research studies (Delaney, 2012). The HIPAA Privacy Rule allows only "covered entities," which include healthcare providers, to "access, use, and disclose identifiable personal health information for treatment, payment and healthcare operations without the need to first obtain a patient's consent" (McGraw, 2012). The Common Rule safeguards privacy by requiring the consent of human research participants and ensuring ethical oversight (Lee, 2009). The first legal issue is that these federal laws attempt to create a distinction between information collection for internal use and information that is intended to contribute to the scientific healthcare community (McGraw, 2012). This means that these laws allow for the extraction of health care information for the purposes of internal quality improvement but not for external publication.

Moreover, because of the interpretation of these federal laws, health care organizations tend to choose not to make clinical data accessible for secondary purposes outside their own internal quality improvement uses (McGraw, 2012). The second legal issue is that organization tend to have a heavy reliance on IRB review. This could introduce selection bias because those who consent to have their information used for research purposes may differ in relevant ways from those who do not consent (McGraw, 2012). The third legal issue is the wide variability among state laws.

Many states have their own privacy laws that are stricter than the federal HIPAA rules. Some states have privacy laws that apply to all health information, while other states have laws that only apply to sensitive information (e.g., HIV test results). Integrating electronic medical records and research becomes a difficult task across healthcare institutions that are subject to different privacy laws (McGraw, 2012).

Proposals have been made to make changes to both HIPAA and the Common Rule governing the research uses of EHR to clarify research rules and processes, which may reduce necessary reliance on IRBs (Delaney, 2012).

To make changes in these federal laws that prevent access to patient information, it is necessary to understand the conceptual ethical framework behind the policy.

Ethical Challenges

These legal challenges arise from ethical concerns regarding human subject research. Three main biomedical ethics principles are used to assess policy regarding research: beneficence, justice, and autonomy (Gostin, 1991). Beneficence, when applied to research, is the principle of promoting the wellbeing of the participants.

However, this means more than simply respecting a patient's wishes. Researchers should maximize the benefits and minimize the risks to human participants. The second principle of justice requires that persons be treated equally unless there is a strong moral reason to do otherwise. Researchers must ensure that participants are not selected based on vulnerability but rather based on factors that are relevant to the problems being studied (Gostin, 1991).

It would be unethical, for example, to do research on homeless people (for a study where homelessness is not relevant) because they are the easiest to exploit. Finally, adhering to the ethical principle of autonomy means respecting a person's individual choices and decision-making processes. This principle requires that all research participation be completely voluntary and not a result of coercion.

Federal regulations on research attempt to address all three of these principles.

However, I will focus only on the HIPAA privacy law, which allows for the sharing of a patient's information only with the patient's consent.

IV. Informed Consent in Research

As mentioned previously, the HIPAA privacy law seeks to respect the ethical principle of autonomy by allowing for the access and use of patient health care information (by non-covered entities) only with the patient's consent. However, receiving consent for large studies can be burdensome and costly, which has prompted some to propose alternative models of consent that are less burdensome (Damschroder, 2007).

In contrast, some have argued that the increased burden of consent does not warrant forgoing the traditional consent process and that policymakers should find other ways to reduce the burden (Elsayyad, 2014).

In the following section, I will outline three different models of receiving patient consent for disclosing access to patient records.

Models of Informed Consent

Opt-In: In this model, patients are provided information about the objectives, risks, burdens, benefits, and alternatives of each study and are asked individually whether they are willing to participate. Although information may be provided in hard copy or electronically, there is typically also personal interaction with a staff member. Under this traditional consent model, a patient may not be enrolled in research without that patient's explicit acknowledgement, usually documented in writing, that the patient has read and understood the information and voluntarily agreed to enroll.

Opt-Out: In this approach, patients are provided with the same information about the objectives, risks, burdens, benefits, and alternatives for each study, which again can be provided in hard copy or electronically. However, unlike the traditional consent model, opt-out information explains that the patient will be enrolled in the study unless the patient specifically requests otherwise. Thus, patients are given study-specific information and a study-specific opportunity to opt out, but expressed prior informed consent is neither solicited nor required.

General/Broad: In this model, patients are informed through stated institutional policies, newsletters, posters in waiting rooms, and patient information sheets that their clinicians and care settings routinely conduct certain types of studies when studies in no way compromise clinical care. Patients are informed of whom to contact with concerns about this policy and may have the option of requesting to be exempted from the policy.

Unlike opt-out consent, there is no disclosure to patients about particular studies and no study-specific opportunity for patients to opt out of participation (Damschroder, 2007).

Perspectives on Informed Consent in Research

Several studies that have investigated patient views on alternative consent models. A study that surveyed Veterans Affairs patients revealed that 74% of respondents preferred an opt-in model, while 26% of respondents preferred an opt-out model of consent for medical research. Of those respondents who chose an opt-out model, 35% preferred a one-time blanket consent, while 39% preferred a traditional consent for each study model (Damschroder, 2007). Other studies have shown that 32.7% of patients (n=597) with some serious genetic or chronic medical condition agreed that researchers should be able to get their medical records without the respondents' permission. When this request was qualified by stating that the database would be set up anonymously, 71% thought that it was a good idea (Kass and Natowicz, 2003). In contrast, the majority of healthy patients (13/17) preferred opt-in consent over broad consent (3/17) and opt-out (1/17) consent (Nair, 2004). Those who were healthy were more likely to prefer an opt-in model than those who were unhealthy, which reveals that health status is a factor that affects patients' opinions on informed consent.

VI. Proposal for Opt-Out Consent for Pragmatic Randomized Research

Observational vs. Experimental Study Designs

The difference between observational and experimental study designs is that, in experimental study designs, "the presence or absence of undergoing an intervention defines the groups" (Song, 2010).

In contrast, in observational studies, there is no intervention; rather, the investigator will observe the relationship between the exposing agent and the disease outcome (Song, 2010). Randomized control trials (RCTs) are a type of experimental study in which participants are assigned randomly to the intervention and placebo groups.

RCTs are known as the highest form of evidence-based medicine (Song, 2010). However, RCTs require a more controlled environment than observational studies, which means that RCTs are very far removed from clinical practice (Hotopf, 2002). Some argue that despite, having good internal validity, they lack external validity, which compromises their utility in applying the conclusions to clinical practice (Hotopf, 2002). Pragmatic randomized controlled trials (PRCTs) seek to provide the best of both worlds: the scientific rigor of RCTs and the external validity of observational studies. PRCTs have several key features: they reflect the heterogeneity of patients in general practice, minimize exclusion criteria, focus on groups with a wide range of diagnoses, define patient groups by presentation rather than diagnosis, may not employ placebos, and may not be blinded (but must carefully conceal allocation during randomization) (Hotopf, 2002).

As a result of PRCTs' middle-of-the-road approach, this makes it a very appealing option for conducting comparative effectiveness research.

Blurring Clinical Care and Clinical Research

The field of research ethics has attempted to analyze how clinical research is fundamentally different from clinical practice (Kass, 2013). However, "drawing a sharp distinction between research and therapy can be appealing, but a growing number of activities in health care cannot be comfortably classified as either research or therapy, the one excluding the other" (Kass, 2013). Participating in a clinical trial, for example, might be the best treatment option for a woman with melanoma (Kass, 2013).

In "The Research-Treatment Distinction: A Problematic Approach for Determining Which Activities Should Have Ethical Oversight," Nancy Kass and her colleagues' proposed that healthcare providers should be allowed to randomize and collect data on medical therapies with similar risk profiles. Because there is no morally relevant difference between clinical care and clinical practice, Kass proposed that we do not distinguish between them. Kass acknowledged that some clinical research undeniably uses an algorithm to determine which intervention that a patient-subject receives.

However, she argued that there is also an element of chance in the treatment options in clinical practice. Kass stated, "Which intervention any given patient will receive in standard practice can be determined by geographic location or hospital catchment area, or by which surgeon they see, than by their health characteristics" (2013).

Kass essentially was commenting on the fact that many medical conditions have multiple effective treatment options. However, because there is little data showing which therapy is the most effective, Kass suggested that, when treatment options have similar risks, healthcare providers should be allowed to randomize the type of therapy given and collect data.

Kass (2013) supported this claim by suggesting that there is often disagreement and, as a result, wide practice variation within the clinical community for various medical interventions.

In "Bioethicists Propose Routine Randomization of Therapy in Clinics", Susan Matthews described how, for many medical conditions, doctors and patients choose from several treatment options approved by the US Food and Drug Administration (FDA).

Matthews explained how Kass's proposal may address the need to assist people to choose amongst a multitude of treatment choices available today. A man diagnosed with prostate cancer is made to select somewhat arbitrarily from surgery, chemotherapy, or monitoring, even though millions of patients before him have already decided on one of these treatment options (Matthews, 253). She commented that, if healthcare institutions had collected outcome data for each patient, doctors might have learned that one approach was the most successful (Matthews, 253).

VII. An Ethical Framework for Opt-Out Randomized Research

We should implement a system of routine randomization of therapies-also known as an opt-out consent for pragmatic randomized trials-that does not simply justify compromising patients' needs for the sake of more generalizable knowledge.

As a result, we should consider at least these four criteria when dealing with the routine randomization of therapies in clinics. I am not arguing that these are the only considerations when dealing with the protection of human subjects in such a scheme, for there may be more considerations. I am arguing that the following four conditions must be minimally met for the routine randomization of therapies to be ethical.

Criterion #1: Randomization Must Not Compromise a Patient's Health and Well-Being

There has been much discussion about the potential conflict between patient care and the standardization of the scientific method (Grunberg, 1387). Jerry Menikoff (2013) stated that "doing research is often going to involve some level of risk to research subjects, risk that is being imposed for a purpose other than for their benefit" (p. S30).

While we have monitoring review boards and regulations dictating the acceptable amount of risk, I would like to focus the discussion on the additional risks that may be imposed by randomization. Imagine the following extreme and unethical example: a man diagnosed with appendicitis by his physician is randomized into a "watchful waiting" intervention group. Because it is known within the medical community that an appendectomy is in fact the best treatment for the patient, it would be unethical for a healthcare system to randomize such interventions for a person diagnosed with appendicitis. I will assume that most will agree that randomization when a particular intervention is known to be so much more effective is unethical.

Now let us turn to another example where the line is not so clear. Imagine a scenario in which a patient has a persistent cough and there are two cough suppressant medications.

Additionally, there is insufficient data on the comparative effectiveness of both drugs. Randomization in this example would satisfy criterion #1 because it is not clear that receiving one specific cough suppressant over another would compromise a patient's health and well-being. The reason that the randomization scenario with the appendectomy is unethical while the randomization scenario with the cough suppressant is ethical is based on whether the patient's health is being compromised by the randomization.

Thus, as long as the randomization scheme does not undeservedly compromise patient health and well-being, it fulfills my first criterion.

Criterion #2: A Patient's Personal Preferences Must Be Accommodated

One issue with clinical research is that patient needs may not be placed first (Kass, 2013). This can be especially problematic because each individual patient has his/her own desires and preferences that may not necessarily align with the drug.

For example, let us imagine a violinist who goes to her primary care physician for an asthmatic condition. Of the three drugs (X, Y, and Z) that are routinely prescribed, one drug is not known to be more effective than either of the other two drugs at treating asthma. However, both drug X and Y have the side effect of mild hand tremors, while drug Z does not. Under a randomization scheme, the violinist has almost a 67% chance of receiving a drug that could cause her hand tremors. Here, the patient has less flexibility to receive a medicine that fits her needs because of the randomization scheme. A randomization scheme that only accounts for drugs with similar effectiveness and does not take personal preferences regarding side effects may infringe on a patient's autonomy over decisions concerning his or her body.

Thus, we should incorporate a randomization system that accommodates patients' personal preferences for other factors than drug effectiveness, such as varying side effects.

Some may argue that the fact that the patient must consent to such randomization automatically fulfills this criterion. They may argue that, if a patient's preference is strong enough, the patient can refuse consent for randomization. While, in this case, providing consent for randomization is necessary, it is not sufficient to meet criterion #2. A process that would fulfill this criterion would be as follows: the physician would have to describe all treatments and all side effects of the treatments. Then, after the patient understands the differences between treatment options (especially differing side effects), then the patient should be asked to consent. Joel Kupersmith's proposal of a simple additional document that only asks for consent randomization would not fulfill this criterion (Kupersmith, 2013, p. S43). It is necessary for the patient to understand fully the relative risks and side effects of each potential treatment option that a patient would randomly receive.

Ultimately, so long as the patient's personal treatment preferences do not call the patient's competence into question, they should be protected and respected. I am hopeful about new research methods that can fulfill this criterion. One such example would be a model implemented by the Clinical Anti-psychotic Trials of Intervention Effectiveness, in which participants may switch to any six "FDA-approved therapies without having to withdraw from the trial based on a clinician's or patient's view that the drug is not working, that the drug is not tolerable or that another drug would be better" (Kass, 2013, p. S11). Therefore, by giving a patient the option to consent to randomly receiving one of the FDA-approved treatment options (while understanding the differences in the risks and side effects of each treatment), we ultimately fulfill this criterion.

Criterion #3: A Patient's Privacy Should Be Respected

My third criterion involves the protection of a patient's privacy.

Normally, in a clinical care setting, patient data are used for the sole purpose of treating the patient. In contrast, for a routine randomization scheme to provide generalizable knowledge, patient data must be recorded and analyzed. We must be particularly careful of protecting the privacy and confidentiality of patient information.

Otherwise, we may risk compromising patient privacy. One concern to keep in mind is the reverse engineering of patient information. We must maintain safeguards to ensure that the details of a patient's illness are stated in a manner that makes it very difficult to identify the patient. I would imagine a system that removes all personal indicators to be sufficient to fulfill criterion #3.

Criterion #4: A Physician Has the Ability to Opt the Patient Out of a Randomized Intervention

Since many clinical research models have a pre-established protocol to assign treatments to research participants, the selection of certain aspects of the treatment regimen is taken out of the hands of the treating physician (Grunberg, 2003). The fact that the physician's judgment is replaced by randomization may lead to less individualized patient care.

I will characterize two types of physician judgment: diagnostic and treatment judgments. With diagnostic judgments, physicians develop a list of differential diagnoses based on a patient's symptoms. This is the type of judgment used when the doctor diagnoses a patient with an illness. The physician's treatment judgment is the decision on which medical intervention is best suited, based on the diagnosis, to treat the patient. Kass's proposal for randomization would decrease the input for physicians' treatment judgments when treatments appear to have similar risk profiles. Some have argued that Kass's proposal would prevent physicians from making intuitive judgments on treatments (Menikoff, 2013, p. S30). While I will not endorse a physician's intuitive treatment judgments in all cases, I will suggest that, at times, it is important for a physician to have the ability to act on his or her judgment.

The reason that we must allow physicians to have the option to opt their patients out of receiving a randomized treatment is to ensure that patients are still able to receive individualized care.

For example, let us imagine an experienced interventional pediatric cardiologist who performs cardiac catheterization on children for the majority of his day five days a week. Because this surgeon is in a sub-subspecialty, has a very particular skill set, and performs the same surgery over and over again, this surgeon will have a clinical sense in performing this surgery.

Subsequently, when there is no academic literature that describes the differences in the effectiveness of surgery approach A versus surgery approach B, I would imagine that the experienced surgeon's judgment would be the patient's best option. I would imagine, similarly, that physicians who have decades of experience with a very specific illness would have a better sense of which treatment is best for a patient based on the patient's individual characteristics. The implication of this is that, if we established a randomization of therapies, we would have to allow the physician to change therapies if he or she believes that the randomized therapy is not working, not tolerable, or inferior to another therapy.

I am not saying that physicians should be able to change therapies simply on a hunch but rather suggesting that we allow physicians to have the opportunity to switch a patient to another intervention after a patient has been randomized to one with adequate justification.

One last consideration is that some will say that some health systems have similar in-house treatment protocols that are not a part of research. These protocols are simply system-wide standards in treating an illness. They would then ask whether these protocols raise the same issues as routine randomization. The answer depends on the circumstances. If the protocols were based on empirical evidence concerning which treatment works best for a certain scenario, then it would appear justifiable to have such protocols (assuming that treatments do not have significant cost differences).

Nonetheless, these protocols should have the flexibility to allow a physician to change a treatment when the physician has reason to believe that another treatment would be best suited for a patient when there is no existing literature comparing treatments. To sum up, criterion #4 is important to provide the opportunity for physicians to provide patients with necessary treatments based on individual characteristics.

VIII. SIGNIFICANCE

Before we can implement the aforementioned proposal, we must survey major stakeholders on their opinions regarding an opt-out randomization proposal. While there is empirical evidence on patient opinions about observational research, as mentioned above, there is very little literature on patients' opinions on informed consent for experimental randomized research. This project provides an opportunity to support health policy decisions regarding informed consent models to better evaluate clinical interventions. Understanding patient opinions regarding the use of clinical data for research is critical to understanding the ethical implications of adopting these alternative informed consent approaches. Patients have the most to gain and the most to lose from this pragmatic comparative effectiveness research.

REFERENCES

Casarett, D. (2000). Determining when quality improvement initiatives should be considered research: Proposed criteria and potential implications. *JAMA: The Journal of the American Medical Association,* 283(17), 2275-2280.

Consumer Reports. (n.d.). *What's behind the ratings-Consumer Reports.* Retrieved from http://www.consumerreports.org/cro/about-us/whats-behind-the-ratings/index.htm.

Damschroder, L. J., Pritts, J. L., Neblo, M. A., Kalarickal, R. J., Creswell, J. W., and Hayward, R. A. (2007). Patients, privacy and trust: Patients' willingness to allow researchers to access their medical records. *Social Science and Medicine*, 64(1), 223-235.

Delaney, B. C., Peterson, K. A., Speedie, S., Taweel, A., Arvanitis, T. N., and Hobbs, F. D. R. (2012). Envisioning a learning health care system: The electronic primary care research network, a case study. *The Annals of Family Medicine*, 10(1), 54-59.

Demaria, A. N. Comparative effectiveness research. *Journal of the American College of Cardiology*, 53(11), 973-975.

Elsayyad, A. S. (2014). Informed consent for comparative effectiveness trials. *New England Journal of Medicine*, 370(issue), 1958-1960.

Faden, R., Kass, N., Whicher, D., Stewart, W., and Tunis, S. (2013). Ethics and informed consent for comparative effectiveness research with prospective electronic clinical data. *Medical Care*, 51, S53-S57.

Godwin, M., Ruhland, L., Casson, I., MacDonald, S., Delva, D., Birtwhistle, R., Lam, M., and Seguin, R. (2014). *Pragmatic controlled clinical trials in primary care: The struggle between external and internal validity. BMC*

Medical Research Methodology, 28(ser. 3). Retrieved from http://www.biomedcentral.com/1471-2288/3/28/

Gostin, L. (1991). Ethical principles for the conduct of human subject research: Population-based research and ethics. *The Journal of Law, Medicine and Ethics*, 19(3-4), 191-201.

Green, L. W. (2006). Public health asks of systems science: To advance our evidence-based practice, can you help us get more practice-based evidence? *American Journal of Public Health*, 96(3), 406-409.

Grunberg, S. M. and Cefalu, W. T. (2003). The integral role of clinical research in clinical care. *New England Journal of Medicine,* 348(14), 1386-1388.

Hotopf, M. (2002). The pragmatic randomised controlled trial. *Advances in Psychiatric Treatment,* 8(5), 326-333.

Kass, N. E., Natowicz, M. R., Hull, S. C., Faden, R. R., Plantinga, L., Gostin, L. O., and Slutsman, J. (2003). The use of medical records in research: What do patients want? *The Journal of Law, Medicine and Ethics*, 31(3), 429-433.

Kass, N. E., Faden, R. R., Goodman, S. R., Pronovost, P., Tunis, S., and Beauchamp, T. (2013). The research-treatment distinction: A problematic approach for determining which activities should have ethical oversight. *Hastings Center Report,* 43(S1), S4-S15.

Kass, N., Faden, R. and Tunis, S. (2012). Addressing low-risk comparative effectiveness research in proposed changes to US federal regulations governing research. *JAMA: The Journal of the American Medical Association*, 307(15), 1589.

Kottow, M. H. (2009). Clinical and research ethics as moral strangers. *Archivum Immunologiae Et Therapiae Experimentalis*, 57(3), 157-164.

Kupersmith, J. (2013). Advances in the research enterprise. *Hastings Center Report*, 43(S1), S43-S44.

Laken, M. A., Dawson, R., Engelman, O., Lovelace, O., Way, C., and Egan, B. M. (2013). Comparative effectiveness research in the 'real' world: Lessons learned in a study of treatment-resistant hypertension. *Journal of the American Society of Hypertension,* 7(1), 95-101.

Lane, J. and Schur, C. (2010). Balancing access to health data and privacy: A review of the issues and approaches for the future. *Health Services Research*, 45(5p2), 1456-1467.

Lee, L. M. and Gostin, L. O. (2009). Ethical collection, storage, and use of public health data: A proposal for a national privacy protection. *JAMA: The Journal of the American Medical Association,* 302(1), 82-84.

Lo, B. and Groman, M. (2003). Oversight of quality improvement: Focusing on benefits and risks. *Archives of Internal Medicine*, 163(12), 1481-1486.

Matthews, S. (2013). Bioethicists propose routine randomization of therapy in clinics. *Nature Medicine,* 19(3), 253.

Mazor, K. M., Sabin, J. E., Goff, S. L., Smith, D. H., Rolnick, S., Roblin, D., ... and Platt, R. (2009). Cluster randomized trials to study the comparative effectiveness of therapeutics: Stakeholders' concerns and recommendations. *Pharmacoepidemiology and Drug Safety,* 18(7), 554-61.

McGraw, D. (2012). *Legal and policy challenges to secondary uses of information from electronic clinical health records*. Retrieved from http:// www.academyhealth.org/files/publications/HIT4AKLegalandPolicy.pdf.

Menikoff, J. (2013). The unbelievable rightness of being in clinical trials. *Hastings Center Report,* 43(S1), S30-S31.

Miriovsky, B. J., Shulman, L. N. and Abernethy, A. P. (2012). Importance of health information technology, electronic health records, and continuously aggregating data to comparative effectiveness research and learning health care. *Journal of Clinical Oncology,* 30(34), 4243-4248.

Morris, M. C. and Nelson, R. M. (2007). Randomized, controlled trials as minimal risk: An ethical analysis. *Critical Care Medicine*, 35(3), 940-944.

Nair, K., Willison, D., Holbrook, A., and Keshavjee, K. (2004). Patients' consent preferences regarding the use of their health information for research purposes: A qualitative study. *Journal of Health Services Research and Policy*, 9(1), 22-27.

Nussbaum, M. C. (2011). *Creating capabilities: The human development approach*. Cambridge, MA: Belknap of Harvard UP.

Olsen, L., Aisner, D. and J McGinnis, J. M. (2007). *The learning healthcare system workshop summary*. Washington, D.C.: The National Academies Press.

Pantalone, K. M., Kattan, M. W., Yu, C., Wells, B. J., Arrigain, S., Jain, A., Atreja, A., and Zimmerman, R. S. (2009). The risk of developing coronary artery disease or congestive heart failure, and overall mortality, in type 2 diabetic patients receiving rosiglitazone, pioglitazone, metformin, or sulfonylureas: A retrospective analysis. *Acta Diabetologica,* 46(2), 145-154.

Peterson, K. A., Fontaine, P. and Speedie, S. (2006). The electronic Primary Care Research Network (ePCRN): A new era in practice-based research. *The Journal of the American Board of Family Medicine*, 19(1), 93-97.

Puglisi, T. (2013). Reform within the common rule? *Hastings Center Report*, 43(S1), S40-S42.

Selby, J. V. and Krumholz, H. M. (2013). Ethical oversight: Serving the best interests of patients. *Hastings Center Report*, S34-S36.

Song, J. W. and Chung, K. C. (2010). Observational studies: Cohort and case-control studies. *Plastic and Reconstructive Surgery*, 126(6), 2234-2242.

Wallace, P. J. (2007). Reshaping cancer learning through the use of health information technology. *Health Affairs*, 26(2), W169-W177.

In: Patient Rights
Editor: Jenna Pope
ISBN: 978-1-63482-136-0

Chapter 3

EFFECTIVE MEDICAL INFORMED CONSENT: A CHALLENGE TO BIOETHICISTS

***David Trafimow*[*,1], *Jordan H. Trafimow*[2] *and A. Jonathan Trafimow*[3]**
[1]New Mexico State University, NM, US
[2]The ARC, Chicago, IL, US
[3]Moritt Hock & Hamroff LLP, NY, US

ABSTRACT

Few would disagree with the desirability of patients providing informed consent before undergoing medical treatments. However, we believe that the obstacles to this goal are more numerous and difficult than bioethicists have realized. Even under ideal circumstances where doctors provide all of the relevant information, a variety of patient limitations may prevent them from using the information properly; in short, patients might be unable to provide *effective* informed consent. In addition, a variety of factors might prevent doctors from providing all of the relevant information in a way that patients can use, or even in any form whatsoever. Finally, we argue that the courts (appropriately) have set legal standards that are lower than ideal bioethical standards, and so legal considerations are capable of providing only the smallest of pushes

* Correspondence to: David Trafimow, Department of Psychology, MSC 3452. New Mexico State University. PO Box 30001. Las Cruces, NM 88003-8001. dtrafimo@nmsu.edu

in the direction of ethical behavior. We challenge the bioethical community to find solutions to all three categories of issues.

Keywords: Informed consent, limitations, medical literacy

According to the American Medical Association (AMA) website (http://www.ama-assn.org/ama/pub/physician-resources/legal-topics/patient-physician-relationship-topics/informed-consent.page), it is both an ethical and legal obligation for doctors to obtain informed consent before performing medical procedures. The website spells out the following:

> "Informed consent is more than simply getting a patient to sign a written consent form. It is a process of communication between a patient and physician that results in the patient's authorization or agreement to undergo a specific medical intervention.
>
> In the communications process, you, as the physician providing or performing the treatment and/or procedure (not a delegated representative), should disclose and discuss with your patient:
>
> - The patient's diagnosis, if known;
> - The nature and purpose of a proposed treatment or procedure;
> - The risks and benefits of a proposed treatment or procedure;
> - Alternatives (regardless of their cost or the extent to which the treatment options are covered by health insurance);
> - The risks and benefits of the alternative treatment or procedure; and
> - The risks and benefits of not receiving or undergoing a treatment or procedure.
>
> In turn, your patient should have an opportunity to ask questions to elicit a better understanding of the treatment or procedure, so that he or she can make an informed decision to proceed or to refuse a particular course of medical intervention."

The AMA website is only one of many sources of information about informed consent. Much has been written about how to ensure that patients are fully informed about their illnesses, potential treatments, and other relevant information (e.g., Merz & Fischhoff, 1990; Paterick et al., 2008; Perry, 1994; Vollman, Winau, & Baron, 1996). Few would disagree that it is better for patients to make informed choices than for them to make uninformed ones. The difficulty is that informed consent involves many tricky issues that the AMA website and other sources do not make immediately obvious, and it is not necessarily clear how to make informed consent happen. Although many bioethicists understand that informed consent, in the sense that the patient knows all relevant information and is able to process all of it effectively, is an ideal goal rather than an achievable goal, we nevertheless believe that there is a tendency to underestimate the problems. Consequently, we have two goals. First, we wish to enumerate the problems so that they are out in the open for everybody to see. Second, despite our pessimism about the likelihood of effective solutions, we hope to stimulate Commentaries where such solutions are proposed. Put more dramatically, we wish to issue a challenge for bioethicists to meet. We would be extremely happy to see our pessimism refuted by the proposal of workable solutions.

PATIENT ISSUES AND LIMITATIONS

There are three sets of interrelated issues and limitations that the serious bioethicist faces when considering how to provide patients with effective informed consent. These pertain to patients, medical providers, and the law. The present section concerns patient issues and limitations, and the subsequent sections address the medical and legal ones, respectively.

Let us pretend, for a moment, that patients know all of the potential positive and negative consequences of all medical options (including no treatment), the probabilities associated with each, and also are rational information processors with unlimited cognitive capacity. Mathematicians, economists, and decision-making researchers have suggested "rational" strategies for deciding what to do, such as to maximize expected utility. This would entail, for each option, to multiply the value of each consequence by its probability, and sum the products across all consequences that might arise $\left(EU = \sum_{i=1}^{N} c_i u_i\right)$. The patient would then choose the option with the largest expected utility. Of course, there are alternative goals that could be considered to be rational, such as minimizing the maximum possible loss (minimax), maximizing the minimum possible gain (maximin), and others. Appropriate equations have been developed that provide rational ways to attain these and other goals that the patient might have.

But alas, patients have limitations that "rational actor" theories ignore. For example, few patients are knowledgeable about the mathematics of decision-making. Even if they possessed all of the relevant information, they would be unlikely to know how to put it together. It has been known for decades that even experts, and especially those who are not experts, generally are unable to use even simple mathematical strategies for properly utilizing information to make optimal decisions (e.g., Gigerenzer & Goldstein, 1996; Goldstein & Gigerenzer, 2002; Kahneman & Tversky, 1979; Tversky & Kahneman, 1974). The issue of patient competency for decision-making has been recognized (Merz & Fischhoff, 1990). For example, Leo (1999) reported that patient competency is an important obstacle to informed consent and also made recommendations for assessing patient competency. In addition, the American Medical Association recognizes that "health literacy" is a problem and they have devoted considerable effort towards addressing it (e.g., see website at http://www.ama-assn.org/ama/pub/about-ama/ama-foundation/our-programs/public-health/health-literacy-program.page).

There also are motivational issues. According to a recent study with 8303 participants, 67% of patients would rather leave the responsibility for the decision up to the doctor (Chung et al., 2012). This relieves the patient from the stress associated with being responsible for making the decision. In addition, having the doctor make the decision reduces the oppressive cognitive demands necessary to carefully consider options, their potential consequences, and probabilities of consequences. Also, the doctor might be seen as an authority figure, and patients may feel that they should comply with authority (e.g., Milgram, 1974). Finally, leaving the decision up to the doctor is a way to prevent arguments with important others, such as family members, friends, and other interested parties; to any argument from an important other, the patient can say, "this is what the doctor recommended." We are not arguing that patients are better off letting doctors make decisions, but it seems unavoidable that many patients have strong motivations in that direction.

Aside from lack of knowledge of the mathematics of decision-making and motivational factors, people have cognitive limitations. If there are many options or potential consequences of options (and relevant probabilities), patients might have insufficient cognitive capacity to process all of them, or even to remember them (e.g., Barrouillet, Lépine, & Camos, 2008; Kahneman, 1973; Vergauwe et al., 2012). Thus, even in the unlikely event that patients are provided with all of the relevant information, know what to do with it, and are motivated to use all of their knowledge, it is likely that cognitive limitations nevertheless will prevent the information from being used optimally.

And then there are a variety of potential distractions. Spouses, friends, children, and others can make demands on patients, whether these demands are implicit or explicit (e.g., Trafimow & Finlay, 1996; Trafimow et al., 2010). Either way, cognitive and motivational capacity devoted to meeting these demands may reduce decision-making capacity. Even if patients do not meet these demands, the process of deciding not to meet them, or dealing with the emotional fallout from not meeting them, can reduce decision-making capacity. It also is possible for others to aid patients in the decision-making process, but on average, our suspicion is that the net effect of others tends to be to reduce decision-making capacity rather than to increase it.

In addition to systematic factors that contribute to poor decision-making, there also are random factors. With the advent of potential performance theory (PPT; Trafimow & Rice, 2008; 2009), psychologists have only recently begun to appreciate the deleterious effects of randomness on decision-making. Based on PPT, much recent research demonstrates that sheer randomness decreases the quality of people's decisions, and prevents them from optimally utilizing even simple information (Rice, Trafimow, & Hunt, 2010; Trafimow & Rice, 2008; 2009). To the extent that randomness enters the process by which patients make medical decisions, and current research suggests that more complexity entails increased randomness (e.g., Rice et al., 2012), the net effect is to reduce the power of patients to make optimal decisions.

Finally, we have thus far glossed over the "values" issue. Even if the doctor explains all of the positive and negative consequences that could arise from all of the possible options, what value should the patient place on each consequence for each option? Suppose that a potential negative consequence of an option is that the patient might get a particular disorder. Well, then, how bad is that disorder? How negative a value should the patient place on the disorder? Is there a cure for the disorder? What is the probability that the cure will be effective? How painful is the cure? Will the cure have its own side effects? If there are side effects (as is usually so), how should the patient assess cures for those side effects? Obviously, there are many more questions that could be asked and so the assignment of values to consequences is not a straightforward matter. Although some of these questions can be addressed by the mathematics of effect sizes (Trafimow, in press), many of them do not have known mathematical solutions. Worse yet, how does one convert a consequence such as "pain" to a number? Much has to be left to subjective judgment that is informed largely by ignorance about medical facts, ignorance about mathematical ways to combine information, the difficulty or impossibility of converting all consequences to numbers, and all of the human biases that have been well documented in the psychological literature (e.g., Gigerenzer & Goldstein, 1996; Goldstein & Gigerenzer, 2002; Kahneman & Tversky, 1979; Tversky & Kahneman, 1974).

Another factor that can influence the values of consequences is effects on third parties. An obvious example might be the effects that abortion has on the potential human, the father, and other interested third parties. In general, family members or caretakers might be affected by treatment options or associated consequences. Even taxpayers might be affected. To the extent that the patient cares about the third parties who are affected by the treatment option chosen, it seems difficult to avoid concluding that at least ideally, patients should be informed about potential third party effects. On the other hand, if the consideration of third party effects leads patients to be more likely to choose treatment options that are not in their best interest, an argument could be made that information about potential third party effects constitutes social pressure to not choose the best option. Does such social pressure imply that the patient isn't really "consenting?" Even if the social pressure issue could be ignored, perhaps information about third party effects increases the likelihood of overwhelming the patient's cognitive capacity, thereby decreasing the patient's ability to make the best possible decision.

In summary, there are many limitations on patients. Even if doctors were to provide all of the relevant information (but see the next section), a variety of factors would prevent patients from being able to use it with optimal effectiveness. It might be possible to argue, in a technical way, that patient limitations are not relevant to the issue of whether they have been completely informed. But it is obvious that patient limitations, whether in terms of knowledge, cognitive capacity, motivational factors, randomness, or the sheer inability to ask and answer all of the relevant questions for assigning values to consequences, renders what we might term "effective informed consent" to be well below that which would be desirable for optimal decision-making. Worse yet, we have thus far assumed something close to perfection with respect to doctors providing relevant information—an assumption that is almost certainly way off the mark, as we address in the subsequent section.

DOCTOR ISSUES AND LIMITATIONS

We have seen that for the patient to make a rational decision, that patient needs to know the treatment options, the potential consequences of each option and how to assign values to them, and the probabilities of the consequences. For many illnesses, this information is known with reasonable precision, and so it is at least within the realm of possibility for the doctor to provide the patient with complete information about the patient's medical condition, prognosis and treatment options. But even under this ideal circumstance there are potential problems. First, even if all of the information is known to medical science, the doctor might not know it. This is particularly true for complex, multi-disciplinary medical situations involving teams of health care providers. Second, the treatment options likely depend on the diagnosis, and the doctor might get the diagnosis wrong or even fail to make one. This is particularly likely if the doctor fails to provide a complete examination, either because of being in a hurry to get to the next patient, because of lack of knowledge, or if multiple diagnoses are needed requiring different medical specialties. Third, the doctor might fail to appreciate the value of information about probabilities of consequences to the patient, or may simply fail to understand how probabilities work at all. As an example of this last, one of the present authors had a conversation with a doctor on birth control and the hypothetical case came up where there are two independent methods of birth control, each of which is 96% effective over the course of a year. What is the probability of pregnancy for the year assuming both methods are used together? The correct answer, of course, is $\big((1-.96)(1-.96)\big) = .0016$ and so the probability of no pregnancy is 1 - .0016 = .9984. The doctor was not even in the ballpark of getting the right answer. Given the display of ignorance about probability, is it realistic to expect this doctor to provide patients with adequate probability information about the consequences of various treatment options, even under the most laudable of intentions?

Aside from knowledge issues, there also are motivational issues. Consider the joke about the guest who complimented the orthopedist on the acquisition of a new yacht and inquired, "How much did it cost?" The orthopedist replied, "Two shoulders and a knee!" Doctors have a financial interest in steering patients towards options that will result in more money for the doctor. Even a well-intentioned doctor might present the treatment options in a way that favors the option that results in the best financial outcome for the doctor (e.g., Berenson, 1987; Hillman, 1987; Hillman, Pauly, & Kerstein, 1989; Stone, 1997).

There also is an interaction between time and financial interest. The less time a doctor spends with each patient, the more patients can be seen, and the result is more money for the doctor. If the doctor spends a lot of time with a particular patient in order to explain clearly all of the options, the potential consequences, and their probabilities, the total time available to treat other patients is reduced. The likely will mean less money for the doctor. Even a doctor unconcerned with money might nevertheless wish to help as many patients as possible, which would suggest that the doctor would wish to see as many patients as possible so as to provide help. Whatever a doctor's reason might be to want to see as many patients as possible, whether due to financial or utilitarian considerations, spending much time to maximize effective informed consent contradicts the goal of seeing as many patients as possible. Given the patient limitations discussed in the foregoing section, providing patients with all of the relevant information, in a way that they can understand and use, might take a prohibitive amount of time, even if it is theoretically possible.

The ability of doctors to provide relevant information to patients depends, in large part, on the information that patients provide to them. Suppose a doctor prescribes a low risk regimen of medicine and the patient skips doses. Or suppose the doctor prescribes a low risk exercise program and the patient fails to perform most of the exercises. If the patient does not improve, and the doctor is not aware that the patient did not follow instructions, the doctor might conclude that the low risk treatment failed. In light of the assumed failure, the doctor might subsequently present potential consequences and probabilities of consequences of riskier treatments in a more favorable light, relative to the low risk treatment that seemingly failed. This can be prevented by simple honesty on the part of the patient who should admit to not following instructions, thereby increasing the accuracy of the information the doctor can provide to the patient.

Even before attempting treatment, patients might fail to provide all of the information the doctor needs to make an accurate diagnosis. For example, for an orthopedist to make a diagnosis, a physical examination is necessary. During the examination, the doctor likely will perform a variety of physical tests, and depend on the patient's ability to say when there is pain and when there is not, and to localize the pain as well as possible. Often, pain cannot be localized very precisely. To the extent that the patient is unable to provide the doctor with precise information during the physical examination, the doctor's diagnosis will become less accurate. Decreased diagnosis accuracy compromises the doctor's ability to provide information the patient needs for effective informed consent.

Issues and Limitations Pertaining to the Law

Court cases addressing informed consent are necessarily concerned with setting standards for determining legal liability, a different issue from establishing ideal ethical norms. Legal standards also vary from state to state.

Nonetheless, in our view, the caution most courts exercise in establishing standards of legal liability either expressly or implicitly recognize many of the limitations on informed consent set forth in this article.

Under New York law, a cause of action for informed consent must allege that "the wrong complained of arose out of some affirmative violation of plaintiff's physical integrity."[1] Failure to advise a patient of the risks of leaving a medical condition untreated does not create legal liability.[2] However, a doctor must inform a patient what he intends to do. The doctor must explain, in words that are understandable to the patient, all the facts that a reasonable medical practitioner would explain regarding (1) the reasonably foreseeable risk which the operation may impose, (2) the patient's existing condition, (3) the purpose and advantages of the operation, (4) the risk involved in not having the operation and (5) the available alternatives, and risks and advantages of same.[3]

California courts have also emphasized a reasonableness standard. In California, "cases have measured the duty to disclose not in terms of an absolute, but as a duty to reveal such information as would be disclosed by a doctor in good standing within the medical community."[4] In probing the contours of the duty of informed consent, the California Supreme Court has identified four "postulates" that frame the duty:

> The first is that patients are generally persons unlearned in the medical sciences and therefore, except in rare cases, courts may safely

---

[1] *Smith v. Fields*, 268 A.D.2d 579, 580 (2d Dep't 2000); *Iazzetta v. Vicenzi*, 200 A.D.2d 209, 212-13 (3rd Dep't 1994).

[2] *Smith*, 268 A.D.2d at 580 ("Since the plaintiff's lack of informed consent claim essentially seeks to recover damages for the defendant's failure to inform her of the risks of allowing periodontal disease to go untreated, it fails to state a cause of action for recovery."); *Campea v. Mitra*, 267 A.D.2d 190 (2d Dep't 1999) ("Here, the plaintiff's claim that the appellant doctor failed to recommend surgery at a time when more beneficial results could have been obtained fails to state a cause of action based on lack of informed consent.")

[3] Public Health Law §2805-d; *Rosado v. Miller*, 2009 N.Y. Misc. LEXIS 330, 2009 N.Y. Slip Op. 50271U (N.Y. Sup. Ct., Kings Cty., Jan. 13, 2009), at *22.

[4] *Cobbs v. Grant*, 502 P.2d 1, 9 (1972). In *Cobbs*, the California Supreme Court also explained that where a doctor "obtains consent of the patient to perform one type of treatment and subsequently performs a substantially different treatment for which consent was not obtained, there is a clear case of battery"; however, "when an undisclosed potential complication results, the occurrence of which was not an integral part of the treatment procedure but merely a known risk," most jurisdictions will not permit the patient to sue for battery, but only for negligence. *Id.* at 7, 8. Although decided more than 40 years ago, the California Supreme Court has subsequently recognized the decision as "one of the epochal opinions in the legal recognition of the medical patient's protectable interest in autonomous decisionmaking." *Arato v. Avedon*, 858 P.2d 598 (1993).

> assume the knowledge of patient and physician are not in parity. The second is that a person of adult years and in sound mind has the right, in the exercise of control over his own body, to determine whether or not to submit to lawful medical treatment. The third is that the patient's consent to treatment, to be effective, must be an informed consent. And the fourth is that the patient, being unlearned in medical sciences, has an abject dependence upon and trust in his physician for the information upon which he relies during the decisional process, thus raising an obligation in the physician that transcends arms-length transactions.

Cobbs, 502 P.2d at 9. From these postulates, the court in *Cobbs* imposed, "as an integral part of the physician's overall obligation to the patient… a duty of reasonable disclosure of the available choices with respect to the proposed therapy and of the dangers inherently and potentially involved in each."[5] Importantly, the court explained, once the risks inherent in a procedure, the risks of not undergoing the treatment and the probability of a successful outcome of the treatment have been explained, "[t]he weighing of these risks against the individual subjective fears and hopes of the patient is… a nonmedical judgment reserved to the patient alone."[6] In California, informed consent also requires disclosure of the material risks resulting from the patient's refusal to consent to a recommended treatment.[7]

The "reasonableness" standard is clearly inconsistent with what we assume to be the objective of most bioethicists: to identify an optimal standard for informed consent, not merely a reasonable one. More than 20 years after the *Cobbs* decision, the California Supreme Court applied the *Cobbs* "reasonableness" standard in *Arato v. Avedon*, 858 P.2d 598 (1993). The facts and the court's analysis in *Arato* provide a useful factual context for assessing the strengths and limitations of the *Cobbs* postulates and approach to informed consent.

In *Arato*, a team of oncologists treated a man with pancreatic cancer. In response to a lengthy questionnaire, the man indicated that he wished to be told the truth about his condition; nonetheless, neither the oncologists nor the

[5] *Cobbs*, 502 P.2d at 10. Other jurisdictions have adopted variations of a reasonableness standard. *See, e.g., Jandre v. Wisconsin Injured Patients*, 813 NW 2d 627 (WI 2012) ("We affirm the decision of the court of appeals by applying the reasonable patient standard (sometimes referred to as the "prudent patient" standard), which Wisconsin has explicitly followed in informed consent cases since at least 1975.")

[6] *Cobbs*, 502 P.2d at 10, 11 (noting an exception to this principle where "it is evident [the patient] cannot evaluate the data, as for example, where there is an emergency or the patient is a child or incompetent" in which case the doctrine of "emergency consent is implied.")

[7] *Truman v. Thomas*, 611 P.2d 902 (1980).

operating surgeon specifically disclosed to him or his wife the high mortality rate associated with pancreatic cancer. The surgeon testified that the patient had "exhibited great anxiety over his condition, so much so that his surgeon determined that it would have been medically inappropriate to disclose specific mortality rates." 858 P.2d at 1177. The oncologists offered a different explanation, essentially testifying that the patient and his wife were told at the outset of the treatment that "most victims of pancreatic cancer die of the disease, that [the patient] was at 'serious' or 'great' risk of a recurrence and that, should the cancer return, his condition would be judged incurable."[8] The oncologists testified that this information was given to the couple "in the context of a series of verbal and behavioral cues designed to invite the patient or family member to follow up with more direct and difficult questions," but that, "in the judgment of his chief oncologist, Mr. Arato, although keenly interested in the clinical significance of the most minute symptom, studiously avoided confronting these ultimate issues; according to his doctors, neither Mr. Arato nor his wife ever asked for information concerning his life expectancy in more than 70 visits over a period of a year."[9] The patient succumbed to his illness, and his wife and two children sued, alleging that the physicians who performed certain procedures (including a pancreas resection and chemotherapy/radiation treatment) "had failed to disclose adequately the shortcomings of the proposed treatment in light of the diagnosis, and thus had failed to obtain the patient's informed consent."[10] The family claimed that, had the deceased known the "bleak truth" regarding his life expectancy, he would have foregone the "unproven therapy" and "live[d] out his last days at peace with his wife and children."[11] The jury ruled for the physicians, but the Court of Appeal ordered a new trial.

In reversing the Court of Appeal and reinstating the jury verdict, the California Supreme Court in *Arato* built upon the *Cobbs* decision. First, the *Arato* court agreed that "each patient presents a separate problem, that the patient's mental and emotional condition is important and in certain cases may be crucial, and that in discussing the element of risk a certain amount of discretion must be employed consistent with the full disclosure of facts necessary to an informed consent."[12] The *Arato* court agreed with *Cobbs* that

---

[8] *Arato,* 858 P.2d at 1178.
[9] *Id.* at 1178.
[10] *Id.* at 1179.
[11] *Id.* at 1179.
[12] *Id.* at 1185 (*quoting Salgo v. Leland Stanford Jr. University Bd. Trustees*, 317 P. 2d 170, 181 (1st Dist. 1957).

informed consent did not require a "minicourse in medical science" or a duty to discuss "relatively minor risks inherent in common procedures"; rather, the critical standard was the patient's need for "adequate information to enable an intelligent choice."[13] This is an inquiry driven by context, warranting deference to the jury's determination.[14] The California Supreme Court expressly declined to "mandate the disclosure of specific information as a matter of law" in favor of requiring "information which the physician knows or should know would be regarded as significant by a reasonable person in the patient's position when deciding to accept or reject a recommended medical procedure."[15] Applying this standard to the facts of a particular case is a function for the jury.[16] To assist the jury, "in an appropriate case, the testimony of medical experts qualified to offer an opinion regarding what, if any, disclosures — in addition to those relating to the risk of death or serious injury and significant potential complications posed by consenting to or declining a proposed treatment — would be made to the patient by a skilled practitioner in the relevant medical community under the circumstances, is relevant and admissible."[17]

The authors find legal considerations to be of limited utility in deriving ethical standards for informed consent. We find ourselves in agreement that the four "postulates" articulated in *Cobbs* are correct and applicable in most situations. We find insightful the tension between the fourth postulate ("that the patient, being unlearned in medical sciences, has an abject dependence upon and trust in his physician for the information upon which he relies during the decisional process") and the court's observation that once the doctor has appropriately explained the medical risks "[t]he weighing of these risks against the individual subjective fears and hopes of the patient is… a nonmedical judgment reserved to the patient alone."

However, there are additional considerations identified in this paper that are not explicitly considered by *Cobbs* or the other cases we reviewed. For example, the *Cobbs* court does not explicitly discuss the possibility that even after the doctor has fully explained the risks of a particular procedure, that the patient still may not understand those risks, and therefore is in no position to

[13] *Id.* at 1186.
[14] *Id.* at 1186.
[15] *Id.* at 1186.
[16] *Id.* at 1187.
[17] *Id.* at 1191.

"weigh" them against the patient's "subjective fears and hopes."[18] Nonetheless, the "reasonableness" standard would appear to absolve the doctor of legal liability under these facts.[19]

At core, however, the legal standards are focused at a different question than this paper considers. The courts (and, where applicable, legislatures) are setting standards for determining legal liability and damages, necessarily a lower standard than the optimal behavior that bioethicists seek to identify.

For example, the bioethicist might reasonably ponder the possibility that, frequently, informed consent is a laudable but ultimately unattainable goal. Complex medical situations may present difficult and constantly changing variables to the patient's prognosis that, quite simply, most patients will not fully understand, and many doctors will be challenged to explain in a cogent manner. Frequently, the patient will do his or her best to understand the situation and treatment alternatives, but, realizing their own limitations (and, perhaps paradoxically, the doctors' limitations as well), will ask the doctor for a recommendation and follow it. If the doctor's explanation was "reasonable" the doctor is unlikely to face legal liability. Nonetheless, it would be inaccurate to conclude that the patient's consent was truly informed.

CONCLUSION

We have suggested that effective informed consent implies not only that the patient has all of the relevant information, but also that the patient is able to use it in a rational way. However, we reviewed several factors that militate against the patient being able to give effective informed consent, even under the assumption that doctors provide all of the relevant information. We also reviewed reasons why doctors often do not provide all of the relevant information. Finally, our brief review of legal cases pertaining to informed consent suggests that the courts are concerned with setting standards for determining legal liability and damages rather than with optimal ethical behavior. Because legal standards for ethical behavior are lower than those that would be set by bioethicists, the courts have provided only a limited impetus towards ethical behavior on the part of doctors and patients. A doctor

---

[18] The patient's ability to understand the doctor's explanation might be impaired for various reasons, such as pain, medication, distraction by other issues such as the stress the patient's condition has placed on loved ones, fear and educational limitations.

[19] The court's explicitly heavy reliance on juries to apply the reasonableness standard, however, permits attorneys ample latitude to second-guess the doctor's explanation.

who adheres only to legal standards traverses only a small proportion of the distance along the pathway to providing the necessary information for effective informed consent.

So where does this leave the bioethicist? As we stated earlier, the goal of obtaining effective informed consent is desirable, but impossible to attain in many circumstances. However, this does not mean that we should "punt on fourth down." Unlike football, where one only has four plays to make a first down and retain possession of the football, there are no such limitations in bioethics. Rather, bioethicists have as many downs as they want. Our hope is that the present article will stimulate others to submit Commentaries that address the particular problems that we mentioned, and propose potential solutions. If each Commentary provides a solution to one problem, the totality of Commentaries will constitute important bioethical progress. Returning to the football analogy, although the bioethical community is unlikely to score a touchdown on a long pass, it might be possible to drive down the field with a succession of short gains.

REFERENCES

Barrouillet, P., Lépine, R., & Camos, V. (2008). Is the influence of working memory capacity on high-level cognition mediated by complexity or resource-dependent elementary processes? *Psychonomic Bulletin & Review*, *15*, 528–534.

Berenson, R. 1987. In a Doctor's Wallet: Financial Confessions of a Sawbones. *New Republic*, 18 May, pp. 11-13.

Chung, G. S., Lawrence, R. E., Curlin, F. A., Arora, V., Meltzer, D. O. (2012). Predictors of hospitalised patients' preferences for physician-directed medical decision-making. *Journal of Medical Ethics*, *38*(2), 77-82.

Gigerenzer, G., & Goldstein, D. G. (1996). Reasoning the fast and frugal way: Models of bounded rationality. *Psychological Review*, *104*, 650–669.

Goldstein, D. G., & Gigerenzer, G. (2002). Models of ecological rationality: The recognition heuristic. *Psychological Review*, *109*, 75-90.

Hillman, A. 1987. Financial incentives for physicians in HMOs: Is there a conflict of interest? *New England Journal of Medicine*, *317*, 1743-1748.

Hillman, A., M. V. Pauly, and J. J. Kerstein. 1989. How do financial incentives affect physicians' clinical decisions and the financial performance of health maintenance organizations? *New England Journal of Medicine*, *321*, 86-92.

Kahneman, D. (1973). *Attention and effort.* Englewood Cliffs, NJ: Prentice-Hall.

Kahneman, D., & Tversky, A. (1979). Intuitive prediction: Biases and corrective procedures. *Management Science, 12*, 313-327.

Leo, R. J. (1999). Competency and the Capacity to Make Treatment Decisions: A Primer for Primary Care Physicians. *The Primary Care Companion to the Clinical Journal of Psychiatry, 1*(5), 131-141.

Merz J. F., & Fischhoff, B. (1990). Informed consent does not mean rational consent: Cognitive limitations on decision-making. *Journal of Legal Medicine, 11*, 321-350.

Milgram, S. (1974). *Obedience to authority.* New York: Harper & Row.

Paterick, T. J., Carson, G. V., Allen, M. C., Paterick, T. E. (2008). Medical informed consent: General considerations for physicians. *Mayo Clinic Proceedings, 83*(3), 313-319.

Perry, C. P. (1994). Conflicts of interest and the physician's duty to inform. *The American Journal of Medicine, 96*(4), 375-380.

Rice, S., Geels, K., Hackett, H., Trafimow, D., McCarley, J. S., Schwark, J. & Hunt, G. (2012). The harder the task, the more inconsistent the performance: A PPT analysis on task difficulty. *Journal of General Psychology, 139*(1), 1-18.

Rice, S. & Trafimow, D., & Hunt, G. (2010). Using PPT to analyze sub-optimal human-automation performance. *Journal of General Psychology, 137*, 310-329.

Stone, D. A. (1997). The doctor as businessman: The changing politics of a cultural icon. *Journal of Health Politics*, Policy and Law, *22*(2), 533-556.

Trafimow, D. (in press). The Ethics of Random Measurement Error in Medical Research: The Problem and the Solution. *The Journal of Bioscience and Medicine.*

Trafimow, D., & Finlay, K. A. (1996). The importance of subjective norms for a minority of people: Between-subjects and within-subjects analyses. *Personality and Social Psychology Bulletin, 22*, 820-828.

Trafimow, D., & Rice, S. (2008). Potential Performance Theory: A general theory of task performance applied to morality. *Psychological Review, 115*(2), 447-462.

Trafimow, D., & Rice, S. (2009). Potential Performance Theory (PPT): Describing a methodology for analyzing task performance. *Behavior Research Methods, 41*(2), 359-371.

Trafimow, D., Clayton, K. D., Sheeran, P., Darwish, A-F. E, & Brown, J. (2010). How do people form behavioral intentions when others have the power to determine social consequences? *Journal of General Psychology, 137,* 287-309.

Tversky, A., & Kahneman, D. (1974). Judgment under uncertainty: Heuristics and biases. *Science*, *185*, 1124-1131.

Vergauwe, E., Dewaele, N., Langerock, N., Barrouillet, P. (2012). Evidence for a central pool of general resources in working memory. *Journal of Cognitive Psychology*, *24*(3), 359-366.

Vollman, T., Winau, R., & Baron, J. H. (1996). History of informed medical consent. *The Lancet*, *347*(8998), 410.

In: Patient Rights
Editor: Jenna Pope
ISBN: 978-1-63482-136-0

Chapter 4

INFORMED CONSENT AND OTHER ETHICAL AND REGULATORY CONSIDERATIONS IN EMERGENCY RESEARCH

Daniel P. Nussbaum, MD and Paul J. Speicher, MD
Duke University Medical Center
Durham, NC, US

ABSTRACT

Complex mechanisms are in place to protect research subjects and to ensure that participants are informed of the risks, benefits, and alternatives available to them prior to enrolling in a research study. However, the process for obtaining informed consent is obscured in the setting of medical emergencies, specifically when subjects are incapacitated. This makes progress in emergency, trauma, and resuscitation research challenging, disciplines in which there is an ongoing need to improve diagnostic and management strategies. There are several guidelines—such as the Declaration of Helsinki, The Common Rule, and the Final Rule—to help researchers navigate this terrain. Unfortunately, none of these regulations sufficiently defines the nuances regarding informed consent among patients in need of emergent intervention. In this chapter, we seek to shed light on the ethical and regulatory considerations surrounding research subjects in emergent medical situations, particularly with regard to the appropriate interpretation of informed consent. As the administrative landscape continues to evolve, principles concerning emergency research should be further standardized to offer sufficient protection to study subjects, while permitting research efforts to proceed without excessive regulatory burden. Throughout this process, it will be crucial for researchers to understand the ethical principles that dictate policy among this uniquely vulnerable population.

INTRODUCTION

Informed consent has played a central role in research ethics since first being conceptualized in the Nuremberg Code of 1947, and later more formalized in the 1950s when the National Institution of Health began requiring it for healthy research subjects. This consent serves as the individual's autonomous authorization of participation in a research study, which often may have limited direct benefit to the participant. Over the past few decades, complex mechanisms have been instituted for the protection of research subjects and to ensure that participants are fully informed of the risks, benefits, and alternatives available to them prior to enrolling in a research study. While there are many established guidelines and requirements to this process, the procedures for properly obtaining informed consent are much less clear in the setting of research during situations of medical emergency, specifically when subjects are incapacitated.

Medical and surgical management in emergency and trauma situations often has, quite literally, life or death consequences. With so much at stake, there is an ongoing need to improve diagnostics and management strategies in these emergent situations. Emergency medical situations, by their very nature, often involve life-threatening conditions and patient populations who are incapable of making decisions. Unfortunately, honoring the core ethical principle of autonomy is often difficult or impossible in these situations, making enrolling patients into research studies an ethical challenge. As there is clearly a need to advance emergency medical and surgical care, the balance between informed consent and advancing medical knowledge must be examined carefully and from multiple perspectives. This chapter is intended to examine the history, ethics, and regulations surrounding emergency research involving adults with life-threatening conditions.

INFORMED CONSENT

Informed consent has existed at the core of biomedical research ethics since the field first began to take shape as an independent discipline. The first article of the Nuremberg Code states: "The voluntary consent of the human subject is absolutely essential." [1] The Code further expands on this, stating that individuals must have sufficient knowledge and comprehension of the elements of the research in question prior to making an affirmative decision to participate as an experimental research subject. Thirty years later, the Belmont Report expanded on this, defining the three "basic ethical principles" of biomedical research: 1. Respect for Persons, 2. Beneficence, and 3. Justice. Belmont specifically addresses informed consent, stating that "Respect for persons requires that subjects, to the degree that they are capable, be given the opportunity to choose what shall or shall not happen to them. This opportunity is provided when adequate standards for informed consent are satisfied." [2] Over the subsequent years, our understanding has evolved further, and most authorities currently define five core components of true informed consent: 1. competence, 2. disclosure, 3. understanding, 4. voluntariness, and 5. actual consent. [3] Unfortunately, none of these landmark documents sufficiently expands on how to address situations in which patients are unable to provide informed consent due to the emergent need for intervention.

PROBLEMS IN EMERGENCY RESEARCH

In the management of critically ill and dying patients, physicians often feel it necessary to attempt non-standard interventions and treatments in attempts to save life or alleviate suffering. Such endeavors are clearly endorsed by the Declaration of Helsinki: "In the treatment of a patient, where proven…therapeutic methods do not exist or have been ineffective, the physician, with informed consent from the patient, must be free to use unproven or new…therapeutic measures, if in the physician's judgment it offers hope of saving life, re-establishing health or alleviating suffering." [4] This provides some justification for research in these individuals, in the form of systematic application of unproven methods in times of dire need. In emergency situations, however, time is often of the essence. Even in patients who are not incapacitated and are technically capable of making decisions, one might argue informed consent is not truly possible. Patients who are aware of their critical situation are almost always in a state of psychological stress, and it is during these times that there exists the least likelihood of full disclosure and understanding, and the greatest threat to voluntariness due to the inherent unbalance present in the doctor-patient relationship.

This is further complicated in situations where patients do not have decision-making capacity and do not have a surrogate decision-maker who might be able to provide consent, as is often the case in emergent medical situations. The Declaration of Helsinki has, in an abstract sense, addressed this concern. Article 29 states that in such situations, research may be done if the condition that prevents consent (i.e., the medical or traumatic insult) is a necessary characteristic of the research population and if research cannot be delayed, the investigator may proceed with the study without informed consent, but must attempt to obtain consent for the subject of a legally authorized representative as soon as possible. [4] The Declaration also clearly mandates that such research be approved by a research ethics committee, but gives little further guidance to such committees regarding the approval process.

EMERGENCY RESEARCH REGULATIONS

Federal regulations regarding research ethics strive to reflect the core guiding principles of Belmont, and are generally summed up what is known as the Common Rule. [5] The Common Rule provides requirements for informed consent, risk thresholds, and the treatment of vulnerable populations. In emergency research involving patients who are capable of providing informed consent, the Common Rule requires that such consent be obtained prior to enrolling the patient in a research study. More importantly, the Common Rule mandates that there is an appropriate balance between the potential benefits of the study and the risks of participation to the subject, and that clinical equipoise must be satisfied for any therapeutic intervention of interest. For patients who are incapable of providing informed consent, the Common Rule mandates that such consent be obtained from a legally authorized representative. However, in situations where there is deemed to be "no more than minimal risk" to participants, the Common Rule provides an exception to the requirement for informed consent. Unfortunately, by its very nature, true emergency research very seldom exposes the patient to only "minimal risk".

Up until the mid-1990s, there were few if any formal mechanisms in place to facilitate obtaining informed consent in the setting of emergency, trauma, and resuscitation research; thus, scientific advancement was dramatically slowed in such areas. By 1993, most experts and regulators believed that by its very nature, clinical research involving life-threatening emergencies could not be performed in agreement with the "minimal risk" requirements stipulated by federal regulations. [6] Because of this, there was—in effect—a moratorium on all trauma and medical resuscitation research in the United States at that time. To address these issues, the DHHS and FDA issued joint regulations permitting certain exceptions from traditional informed consent requirements in studies of emergent and life threatening conditions. These exceptions have become colloquially known as the Final Rule, and provide a regulatory definition of emergency research and when it is considered exempt:

> "These investigations involve human subjects who have a life-threatening medical condition that necessitates urgent intervention (for which available treatments are unproven or unsatisfactory), and who, because of their condition (e.g., traumatic brain injury) cannot provide informed consent. The research must have the prospect of direct benefit to the patient and must involve an investigational product that, to be effective, must be administered before informed consent from the subject or the subject's legally authorized representative can be obtained and in which there is no reasonable way to identify prospectively individuals likely to become eligible for participation." [7]

The Final Rule may only be applied in situations of life-threatening emergency medical conditions, and must have the potential to directly benefit study participants. In addition to defining the acceptable risks and required benefits of such research, the Final Rule also outlines requirements for disclosure of the study to the community, and mandates that study investigators consult with the community and integrate the community's concerns into the IRB review process.

ETHICAL CONSIDERATIONS AND DILEMMAS

While regulations have attempted to clarify the extent to which emergency research can be conducted in individuals both with and without decision-making capacity to provide informed consent, the ethical nuances have yet to be resolved. Regarding the acceptable risk balance, the Final Rule states that permissible risk is that which is "reasonable in relation to what is known about the medical condition of the potential class of subjects [and] the risks and benefits of standard therapy". This statement, however, seems to indicate that there is no upper limit on the extent of permissible risk to which a study may subject its participants, so long as the clinical status of the participant is sufficiently grim. To many this may be a reasonable proposition: as the likelihood of imminent death or severe disability increases, so does the acceptable risk. Unfortunately, this framework is at odds with the basic ethical principle of respect for persons from Belmont and the implications for informed consent. This provision states that vulnerable subjects, which these individuals certainly are, must be protected from risk in concordance with the magnitude of their vulnerability, which in many ways is the antithesis of the guidelines provided by the Final Rule.

Similarly, while community involvement is a clearly-defined requirement per the Final Rule, what this means—and the ethical implications—have not been clearly established. Often times this is executed in the form of public meetings and the addition of laypeople within the community to the IRB. Oftentimes, this is interpreted as a need to proactively seek out individuals from the community who are part of a similar risk-profile demographic as those who would be the subjects of the anticipated research project. The investigator would then take a random cross-sectional sample of this population, describing the study objectives and asking if the individual would be willing to participate if in such a situation. Doing this, however, triggers important ethical considerations of how properly to identify the community to be consulted, and what the best methods of disclosure and discussion are. Furthermore, community consultation may not adequately nor directly address protections of the individual, which are at the core of research ethics and regulations.

CONCLUSION

Conducting research on patients in the setting of emergent medical conditions is fraught with ethical and regulatory considerations, particularly surrounding the appropriate interpretation of informed consent. Researchers must navigate a particularly grueling set of contradictory federal regulations and ethical frameworks, all while attempting to study unproven diagnostic modalities and interventions in some of the sickest patients seen in medical practice. As the regulatory landscape will almost certainly continue to evolve over the coming decades, researchers must maintain the ability to navigate regulatory barriers while always—as their primary concern—protecting the individual from undue risk. In the future, regulations regarding emergency research should be further standardized to offer sufficient protection to study subjects while still permitting critically important emergency research efforts to proceed without excessive regulatory burden.

REFERENCES

[1] "Trials of War Criminals before the Nuremberg Military Tribunals under Control Council Law No. 10", Vol. 2, pp. 181-182. Washington, D.C.: U.S. Government Printing Office, 1949.

[2] National Commission for the Protection of Human Subjects of Biomedical and Behavioral Research. The Belmont Report: Ethical Principles and Guidelines for the Protection of Human Subjects of Research. Washington, DC: Government Printing Office, 1979.

[3] Meisel A, Roth LH. What we do and do not know about informed consent. *JAMA*. 1981 Nov 27;246(21):2473-7

[4] Declaration of Helsinki World Medical Association. Available from: http://www.wma.net/en/20activities/10ethics/10helsinki/[accessed on 25 March 2014].

[5] Department of Health and Human Services. Rules and regulations: Protection of human subjects. Title 45, code of federal regulations, part 46. *Fed Regist.* 1991; 56:28003.

[6] McRae A, Weijer C. U.S. Federal Regulations for emergency research: a practical guide and commentary. Acad Emerg Med. 2008;15(1):88-97.

[7] Food and Drug Administration. Title 21 CFR 50.24. Exception from informed consent requirements for emergency research. *Fed Regist.* 1996; 61:51528.

In: Patient Rights
Editor: Jenna Pope

ISBN: 978-1-63482-136-0

Chapter 5

RIGHT TO HEALTH AND DENTAL CARE

Francesca Zangari, MD*

Dental Service - Local Health Service of Romagna, Italy

ABSTRACT

Universal access to oral health care is a fundamental right for everyone and the primary purpose of all health care professionals, organizations, and public policy should be to improve oral health. In today's economic climate, health care systems are challenged by the need to prioritise and address the inequitable distribution of resources in society. Market forces, scarcity of funding, and lack of clarity as to who is responsible for ensuring that oral care is available add to these difficulties. Dentistry is not part of the universal health care system in all countries: inequalities within dentistry are common and reflected in wide differences in the levels of oral health and the standard of care available both within and between countries and communities. Oral health care is complex and there is no consensus within the profession about what counts as normal human functioning and little consensus about what basic needs entail especially where resources are limited. Moreover, vulnerable populations are often further disadvantaged by physical dis-abilities, illness, poverty, and other socio-economic conditions that impede their access to care. Improving access to oral health care is a social problem intimately intertwined with general health care access, education, and oral health literacy of the public, employment, insurance,

* Corresponding author: Francesca Zangari, MD. E-mail: f.zangari@tin.it.

and a host of other societal factors. The dental professions will not solve these problems in isolation: a systematic approach is essential if we are to understand, evaluate, and institute structural, organizational, professional, and individual change in the oral health delivery system.

1. HEALTH AND DENTAL CARE

Health care, including dental care, is a social good and a fundamental right for everyone. In today's economic climate, health care systems are challenged by the need to prioritise and address the inequitable distribution of resources in society. Market forces, scarcity of funding, and lack of clarity as to who is responsible for ensuring that oral care is available add to these difficulties. Moreover, vulnerable populations are often further disadvantaged by physical disabilities, illness, poverty, and other socio-economic conditions that impede their access to care. Vulnerable populations tend to experience worse health outcomes, face barriers to care, have higher rates of morbidity and mortality than the general population, and have little or no control over the conditions that contribute to their situation. There are groups of people who, because of financial circumstances, are unable to access basic health care. In particular, poor oral health affects one's general health and further disadvantages people from securing jobs and trying to live a decent life.

Health care, including dental care, is a social good and a fundamental right for everyone. Oral health is a component of overall health, and oral illness is associated with several adverse health effects [1]. In meta-analyses, periodontitis (i.e., chronic inflammation of structures that hold the tooth) has been associated with coronary heart disease [2], respiratory disease [3], and preterm birth [4] – although the evidence remains weak due to a limited number of low quality studies. Dental disease has also been linked to chronic medical illnesses [5], as well as to functional, social and psychological limitations [6]. There is a growing body of literature linking oral illness to chronic medical conditions such as type II diabetes, osteoporosis, Alzheimer's disease and cognitive functioning [7-11]. So, oral health problems, like other health problems, can limit a person's activity, participation in the workforce, quality of life and mental health [12]. Moreover, there are groups of people who, because of financial circumstances, are unable to access basic health and dental care. Income-related inequity in oral health has been well established both globally [13] with higher levels of dental disease being concentrated among those with lower incomes and lower socio-economic status [14, 15].

The consequence is that vulnerable populations, often further disadvantaged by physical disabilities, illness, poverty, and other socio-economic conditions that impede their access to care, tend to experience worse health outcomes, face barriers to care, have higher rates of morbidity and mortality than the general population, and have little or no control over the conditions that contribute to their situation.

To limit the access of indigent people who need health care appears contrary to the mission of health professionals and providers, when the primary aim of oral health delivery systems should be to deliver effective and efficient care while respecting patient dignity and autonomy, according to the precepts and definition of the profession and providers.

2. Access to Dental Care

When a person attends a dental practice requiring dental treatment, the process the person becoming a patient begins and this journey from person to patient involves four steps: acceptance, diagnosis, treatment, and payment. Acceptance begins when health professionals honor an ethical responsibility to talk with persons who have asked for help and engage them in dialogue related to their health and, if necessary, help to ensure some mechanism by which they can access care. Acceptance is a normative ethical principle centrally related to the applied ethical issue of access to care.

Accepting, talking to, and guiding patients might seem to be a simple practice, one that ethicists and health providers likely presuppose and believe they already adhere to and accomplish. However, acceptance may not be so transparent or manifest, as demonstrated by health providers who seem to engage in various styles of acceptance that result in the creation of barriers to access.

The three basic types and styles of acceptance are random, selective, and universal [16]. Random acceptance is practiced when providers do not specifically plan their actions to determine which persons will be seen for discussion and perhaps treated. Surgery location, hours of operation and languages spoken are types of actions that contribute to patterns of random patient acceptance, which nonetheless result in the unintentional exclusion of patients. For example, a surgery that is wheelchair-inaccessible leads to exclusion and reduces access to care. Selective acceptance is an intentional process that specifically seeks to limit who can be seen and treated. Patient selection can be based on finances and ability to pay, on employer or insurance groupings. All such acts result in the intentional, selective acceptance of some patients and the exclusion of others. As long as barriers created by random and selective acceptance continues, injustice and reduced access to care will persist and prevent people from being accepted for discussion about their possible treatment needs. On the contrary, universal acceptance intends to remove barriers that accidentally or intentionally keep people from being accepted for a dialogue with a health care professional [17]. Universal access to oral health care is a fundamental right for everyone and the primary purpose of all health care professionals, organizations, and public policy should be to improve oral health.

Since oral health is an essential aspect of general health, ensuring equity in oral health care is as important as ensuring equity in other forms of health care [18]. However, global oral health disparities persist and their evidence (i.e., lower socioeconomic status being associated with greater oral disease) is well documented [19, 20], both in general adult and elderly populations [21-23]. Every society, especially the complex societies of the contemporary world, has a system of social structures by which it manages the distribution of its resources among the individuals and groups that make up the society. Whenever a society is establishing or modifying one of these systems, one unavoidable question in a world of finite resources is the ethical question of how to prioritize the various benefits the society's people will have access to or will fail to have access to by means of these systems. Because certain kinds of human need have special ethical importance, the distribution systems should be so designed that everyone in the society can meet these needs, i.e., that providing everyone in the society access to the resources they require to meet these special needs must be one of the society's highest ethical priorities. Dentistry is not part of the universal health care system in all countries. Inequalities within dentistry are common and are reflected in wide differences in the levels of oral health and the standard of care available both within and between countries and communities. The World Health Organization (WHO) has called for the reduction of inequity in oral health as one of its major worldwide goals [24]. With respect to the use of dental care, considerable socioeconomic inequalities at both the individual (intra-country) and collective (inter-country) levels across Europe and worldwide has been reported [13, 25]. Public service, where it exists, is mostly inadequate with regard to the means and human resources to treat all segments of the population. Even when dental care is limited to particular conditions of vulnerability, sanitary (conditions of sanitary kind which make dental treatments essential or necessary) or social (conditions of social and economic disadvantage generally related to the low income and/or to marginally or social exclusion which prevent access to private dental treatments), patients have access problems related tounder-provision or waiting lists etc. Moreover, because of lack of resources, not all dental treatments are guaranteed in the public health care: often dentures implants are excluded and only emergency treatment is provided.

There is an ethical professional duty based on our social contract to provide limited case to relieve pain and suffering, keeping in mind that pain and sepsis and any other conditions that prevent or severely limit normal nutrition and speech should take priority [26]. But, it is not easy to define what 'basic' oral health care entails: oral health care is too complex and depends too much on the clinical details of the patient's conditions that no consensus exists within the profession about what counts as normal human functioning and little consensus about what basic needs entail especially where resources are limited. In addition, differences exist regarding the ways in which the quality of dental care is monitored: by control department, administrative body, or profession; sometimes, by patient complaints, when a formal direct control does not exist. In many countries, dentistry is still mostly a fee-for-service system and private, favouring wealthier patients and those with dental insurance [27]. The role of dental insurance and other third-party payers, including government dental care programs, is now increasing.

The insurance payment limits by itself the access to oral health care: patients can choose basic care insurance package and decide to pay more, if they can, for adding all other dental care they need; moreover, third party payers typically limit the treatments that are covered for a given diagnosis, although those treatments covered are within the recognized standard of care for that diagnosis.

Some third-party payers are profit-making corporations that limit treatments to the least expensive precisely for the sake of market success for the corporation. This is in comparison with government programs and some not-for profit organizations that limit costly treatments from a conscientious effort to ration limited resources equitably across a disadvantage population of oral health patients. Income-related inequality in need for dental care exists even in the presence of dental insurance coverage and good dental hygiene habits. These findings highlight the need for increased access to dental care for low-income populations and families living in poverty.

While the conceptual model for oral health inequalities is complex, differential access to dental care may contribute to oral health disparities, given that forgoing dental care due to financial hardship is associated with poorer oral health [28-33].

CONCLUSION

Full access to care is a multidimensional phenomenon and requires multidisciplinary support from many parts of society and a reform of existing public policy, law, and financing. The problem of inadequate access to dental care for the underserved segments of the population is still complex and cannot be solved easily or quickly.

A single, simple solution will not be effective and, generally, the "one size fits all" concept will generate inadequate solutions. It is imperative that the specific barriers to care for each group are identified and understood. Programs designed to promote improved access must adequately address the problems that are identified if access is to be achieved.

Improving access to oral health care is a social problem intimately intertwined with general health care access, education, and oral health literacy of the public, employment, insurance, and a host of other societal factors. The dental professions will not solve these problems in isolation: a systematic approach is essential if we are to understand, evaluate, and institute structural, organizational, professional, and individual change in the oral health delivery system. Dentistry runs the risk that the public perceptions of the oral health professions is that they respond mainly to consumers' desires rather than to patients' needs. Improving access to oral health care is not the dental profession's sole responsibility. It is a societal problem intimately intertwined with general health care access, education, and oral health literacy of the public, employment, insurance, and a host of other societal factors. A systematic approach is essential if we are to understand, evaluate, and institute structural, organizational, professional, and individual change in the oral health delivery system. The oral health professions and their members can do a great deal to help bring about the social dialogue that will be necessary to change the social systems that control access to oral health care in our society. The effort should engage the schools of dentistry and dental hygiene and other educational institutions in the oral health community to not only support this message, but to directly educate their students about it in all its subtlety in order to secure the message within the oral health community for years to come. And there are also other potential allies in the oral health community—manufacturers, insurers, advertisers, management consultants, laboratories, owners of large practice settings, etc., that can help to lead to a genuinely shared commitment within the oral health professions to take more effective action, in the hope that oral health care might become more readily accessible to everyone.

REFERENCES

[1] Chapple, I. L.: The impact of oral disease upon systemic health-symposium overview. *J. Dent.* 2009, 37(8):S568-S571.

[2] Bahekar, A. A., Singh, S., Saha, S., Molnar, J., Arora, R.: The prevalence and incidence of coronary heart disease is significantly increased in periodontitis: a meta-analysis. *Am. Heart J.* 2007, 154(5): 830-837.

[3] Scannapieco, F. A., Bush, R. B., Paju, S.: Associations between periodontal disease and risk for nosocomial bacterial pneumonia and chronic obstructive pulmonary disease. A systematic review. *Ann. Periodontol.* 2003, 8(1):54-69.

[4] Vergnes, J. N., Sixou, M.: Preterm low birth weight and maternal periodontal status: a meta-analysis. *Am. J. Obstet. Gynecol.* 2007, 196 (2): 135 e131-137.

[5] Cooney, P. Preface to the Canadian Health Measures Survey results – oral health statistics, 2007-2009. *Chronic Diseases in Canada*. 2010; 30 (4):115-116.

[6] Locker, D., Matear, D. *Oral disorders, systemic health, well being and the quality of life - A summary of recent research evidence.* Community Health Services Research Unit, Faculty of Dentistry, University of Toronto. [Accessed 2014 Jan. 28]. Available:http://s3.amazonaws.com/zanran_storage/www.utoronto.ca/ContentPages/9519770.pdf.

[7] Preshaw, P. M., Bissett, S. M.: Periodontitis: oral complication of diabetes. *Endocrinol. Metab. Clin. N. Am.* 2013, 42(4):849-867.

[8] Kamer, A. R., Craig, R. G., Dasanayake, A. P., Brys, M., Glodzik-Sobanska, L., de Leon, M. J.: Inflammation and Alzheimer's disease: possible role of periodontal diseases. *Alzheimers Dement.* 2008, 4(4): 242-250.

[9] Passos, J. S., Vianna, M. I., Gomes-Filho, I. S., Cruz, S. S., Barreto, M. L., Adan, L., Rosing, C. K., Cerqueira, E. M., Trindade, S. C., Coelho, J. M.: Osteoporosis/osteopenia as an independent factor associated with periodontitis in postmenopausal women: a case-control study. *Osteoporos. Int.* 2013, 24(4):1275-1283.

[10] Sandberg, G. E., Sundberg, H. E., Fjellstrom, C. A., Wikblad, K. F.: Type 2 diabetes and oral health: a comparison between diabetic and non-diabetic subjects. *Diabetes Res. Clin. Pract.* 2000, 50(1):27-34.

[11] Listl, S.: Oral health conditions and cognitive functioning in middle and later adulthood. *BMC Oral Health* 2014, 14:70. doi: 10.1186/1472-6831-14-70.

[12] Gift, H. C., Atchison, K. A. Oral health, health, and health-related quality of life. *Med. Care*. 1995; 33 (11 Suppl.): NS57-77.

[13] Hosseinpoor, A. R., Itani, L., Petersen, P. E.: Socio-economic inequality in oral healthcare coverage: results from the World Health Survey. *J. Dent. Res.* 2012, 91(3):275-281.

[14] Snow, P., McNally, M. E. Examining the implications of dental treatment costs for low-income families. *J. Can. Dent. Assoc*. 2010;76 (2):a28.

[15] Sabbah, W., Tsakos, G., Chandola, T., Sheiham, A., Watt, R. G. Social gradients in oral and general health. *J. Dent. Res*. 2007; 86(10):992-996.

[16] Corsino, B. V., Patthoff, D. E. Jr. The Ethical and Practical Aspects of Acceptance and Universal Patient Acceptance. *J. Dent. Educ*. 2006; 70 (11): 1198-1201.

[17] Werhane, P. Access, Responsibility, and Funding: A Systems Thinking Approach to Universal Access to Oral Health. *J. Dent. Educ*. 2006; 70 (11): 1184-1195.

[18] Heymann, J., Cassola, A., Raub, A., Mishra, L. Constitutional rights to health, public health and medical care: The status of health protections in 191 countries. *Glob. Public Health* 2013; 8(6): 639-653. doi:10.1080/17441692.2013.810765.

[19] Watt, R., Sheiham, A.: Inequalities in oral health: a review of the evidence and recommendations for action. *Br. Dent. J*. 1999, 187(1):6-12.

[20] Guarnizo-Herreno, C. C., Watt, R. G., Fuller, E., Steele, J. G., Shen, J., Morris, S., Wildman, J., Tsakos, G.: Socioeconomic position and subjective oral health: findings for the adult population in England, Wales and Northern Ireland. *BMC Public Health* 2014, 14:827. doi: 10.1186/1471-2458-14-827.

[21] Listl, S.: Income-related inequalities in denture-wearing by Europeans aged 50 and above. *Gerodontology* 2012, 29(2):e948-e955.

[22] Listl, S., Moran, V., Maurer, J., Faggion, C. M. Jr: Dental service utilization by Europeans aged 50 plus. *Community Dent. Oral Epidemiol.* 2012, 40(2):164-174.

[23] Listl, S.: Income-related inequalities in dental service utilization by Europeans aged 50+. *J. Dent. Res*. 2011, 90(6):717-723.

[24] Petersen, P. E.: The World Oral Health Report 2003: continuous improvement of oral health in the 21st century–the approach of theWHO Global Oral Health Programme. *Community Dent. Oral Epidemiol.* 2003; 31(Suppl. 1):3-23.

[25] Tchicaya, A., Lorentz, N.: Socioeconomic inequalities in the non-use of dental care in Europe. *Int. J. Equity Health* 2014; 13(1):7. doi: 10.1186/ 1475-9276-13-7.

[26] Ozar, D. T. Basic Oral Health Needs: A Public Priority. *J. Dent. Educ.* 2006; 70(11): 1159-1165.

[27] Dharamsi, S., Pratt, D., MacEntee, M. How Dentists Account for Social Responsibility: Economic Imperatives and Professional Obligations. *J. Dent. Educ.* 2007; 71(12): 1583-1592.

[28] Azogui-Lévy, S., Rochereau, T. Comportements de recours aux soins et santé bucco-dentaire. IRDES 2005.

[29] Sanders, A. E., Spencer, A. J., Slade, G. D.: Evaluating the role of dental behaviour in oral health inequalities. *Community Dent. Oral Epidemiol.* 2006; 34(1):71-79.

[30] Ramraj, C., Quinonez, C. R.: Self-reported cost-prohibitive dental care needs among Canadians. *Int. J. Dent. Hyg.* 2013; 11(2):115-120.

[31] Thompson, B., Cooney, P., Lawrence, H., Ravaghi, V., Quinonez, C.: The potential oral health impact of cost barriers to dental care: findings from a Canadian population-based study. *BMC Oral Health* 2014, 14:78. doi: 10.1186/1472-6831-14-78.

[32] Baelum, V., van Palenstein Helderman, W., Hugoson, A., Yee, R., Fejerskov, O.: A global perspective on changes in the burden of caries and periodontitis: implications for dentistry. *J. Oral Rehabil.* 2007; 34 (12):872-906.

[33] Pegon-Machat, E., Tubert-Jeannin, S., Loignon, C., Landry, A., Bedos, C.: Dentists' experience with low-income patients benefiting from a public insurance program. *Eur. J. Oral Sci.* 2009; 117(4):398-406.

In: Patient Rights
Editor: Jenna Pope

ISBN: 978-1-63482-136-0

Chapter 6

The Ethics of HIV Screening Targeted to the Seriously Mentally Ill

Mary V. Seeman*, OC, MDCM, FRCPC, FACP, DSc
Department of Psychiatry, University of Toronto, Canada

Abstract

Background: There is a higher than expected global prevalence of HIV risk behavior among adults with severe mental illness (SMI) and a consequently high HIV prevalence. The US Center for Disease Control recommends yearly HIV testing of high-risk groups but the SMI population is rarely tested.

Objective: This paper discusses the pros and cons of provider-initiated screening for HIV in mental health settings that serve the seriously mentally ill. Method: A literature review of the ethics of HIV screening as it pertains to the seriously mentally ill.

Results: There are several benefits to provider-initiated HIV screening of SMI patients in mental health settings. It motivates risk reduction behavior when accompanied by pretest and posttest counseling. Individuals who test positive obtain immediate access to ongoing medical care for HIV. The public health benefit is that at risk individuals modify their behavior and thus reduce incidence rates while HIV+ individuals obtain treatment that renders them less infectious, further driving down

* mary.seeman@utoronto.ca; Professor Emerita

infection rates. There are ethical issues, however, that need to be addressed. Does targeting SMI individuals increase their stigmatization? Can provider-initiated screening be considered voluntary? Is consent in this cognitively challenged population truly informed? Do perceived incentives negate the voluntary aspect of consent? Can confidentiality be guaranteed in a mental health setting where service users constantly interact? Whose responsibility is it if HIV+ persons fail to disclose their status to sexual partners or fail to reduce risk behaviors? Does the public health benefit outweigh individual benefit? Is there a financial cost benefit?

Conclusion: Ethical issues are important to consider and discuss. Safeguards need to be in place. On the whole, however, this paper endorses the provision of HIV screening in mental health settings for the seriously mentally ill.

Keywords: Serious mental illness, HIV screening, consent, voluntariness, privacy, disclosure

The seriously mentally ill (SMI), defined by severity of psychotic symptoms, duration of illness, and functional disability, comprise approximately 2.8% of the US population [1], most of whom are in continuous or intermittent treatment. Among these patients, there is a high prevalence of HIV risk behavior [2] involving multiple, relatively unknown sexual partners, unprotected sexual activity, untreated sexually transmitted disease, and the use of injection drugs). This translates into a relatively high prevalence of HIV infection. In the USA, prevalence rates in mentally ill patients in general have been reported to be 5 - 23%, compared with 0.3 - 0.4% in the general population [3]. Rates change over time and the specifics of the population studied. In a recent study, rates among those with SMI were found to be at least four times higher than the national average [4]**.** The prevalence appears to be highest among individuals with SMI who also suffer from a substance abuse disorder [5].

In 2006, the US Center for Disease Control recommended yearly HIV testing of high-risk groups [6], but the SMI population is not routinely tested [7]. A 2009 review found that, in any given year, fewer than half (17%–48%) of SMI patients were ever tested [8].

This paper discusses the pros and cons of provider-initiated screening for HIV in mental health settings that serve the seriously mentally ill. Method: The following search terms: 'Serious/severe mental illness'; 'HIV screening'; 'HIV test'; 'ethics'; 'consent'; 'opt in'; opt out'; 'confidentiality'; 'decisional capacity'; 'privacy'; 'voluntary'; 'justice'; 'mandatory'; 'stigma'; 'incentives'; 'risk'; 'benefit'; 'treatment access' were entered into Google Scholar in a variety of combinations. Articles in English were explored from the year 2000 till the present, searching for ethical concerns related to HIV screening in the SMI population.

PROVIDER-INITIATED HIV SCREENING IN MENTAL HEALTH SERVICES

Because approximately 25% of Americans who are HIV positive are unaware of the fact and, as a consequence, fail to seek early intervention, thus jeopardizing their personal health and posing a risk of infection to others, the Centers for Disease Control (CDC) has argued that HIV testing should be routinely offered in all healthcare settings. According to the CDC, general consent for medical care should encompass consent for blood tests, including a test for HIV [9]. In the late 1980s, when there was no treatment for HIV and when persons with HIV were stigmatized and discriminated against, the case was made for not offering HIV tests but, instead, waiting for individuals to volunteer to have them done. And, even then, to provide extensive pre and post test counseling. The situation has markedly changed since that time. HIV has become a chronic infection, still stigmatized, but far less than it was 30 years ago. Treatment is available and effective as long as it is indefinitely maintained. Treated individuals are significantly less infectious than those who are untreated [10] so that there is a known public health, as well as individual health, advantage to ascertaining and treating everyone who is affected. In view of the current situation, what are the ethical challenges to provider-initiated HIV screening of the seriously mentally ill in mental health services?

STIGMA LAYERING

Substantial stigma (enacted stigma, perceived stigma, self-stigma) continues to exist against those with mental illness and also against those infected with HIV based on the mistaken belief that these illnesses are brought about by immoral or irresponsible conduct, and reinforced by the fear that both mental illness and HIV are, in different ways, contagious. In 2003, it was reported that more than one-third of participants in a survey were concerned about being tested for HIV because of AIDS-associated stigmatization [11]. Such concerns argue against targeting mental health populations in HIV screening for fear of adding another layer of discrimination on a group that is already vulnerable and already stigmatized [12].

The routine testing of pregnant women, for instance, has been opposed because an HIV+ woman could be accused of promiscuity and at risk for enacted stigma in the form of sexual partner violence [13]. The same would hold true for vulnerable mental health patients, both men and women. In the case of SMI patients, not only sexual partners, but family members such as caretaking parents might react negatively to a positive HIV test and potentially retaliate against the patient. Since SMI patients are often financially and emotionally dependent on family members, this is an important consideration. In the case of SMI patients living in a communal residence or boarding home, the potential reaction of landlords and co-residents to a positive HIV test may also be critical. Employers need to be considered as well. Employment is always tenuous in the SMI population and loss of hard won employment may become a reality in the face of an employer learning of a positive test. Healthcare personnel may themselves not be immune to stigmatizing reactions. A national survey of 43 community-based AIDS service organizations have reported that a large number of nursing homes and psychiatric facilities in large metropolitan areas refused to accept clients infected with HIV [14]. A national study of 2466 HIV-infected adults receiving care in the United States showed that 25% thought that their clinicians discriminated against them when their HIV test came back positive [15]. Because an HIV diagnosis is traumatic [16], stigmatizing attitudes may be perceived by the affected person even when no actions are taken by others. Self-stigma in the form of lowered self-esteem; isolation, and social avoidance often result. This is an added burden on SMI patients. It can also be argued, however, that by making HIV testing routine, the stigma attached to HIV is reduced. Several studies report a convincing association between reduced levels of perceived stigma and testing for HIV as long as pre and post test counseling is in place [17-19].

VOLUNTARINESS

Although mandatory HIV screening has, on occasion, been considered [20,21], it is generally regarded as overly paternalistic and a violation of consent and privacy ethics [22]. Provider-initiated screening is voluntary.

After being provided with comprehensive pre-test information, patients are given the opportunity to sign up for it (opt in) or to refuse it (opt out).

The ethical question in a mental health setting is whether SMI patients possess a sufficient degree of agency to allow them to either opt in or to opt out [23,24]. They may have inadequate knowledge and understanding of the risk situation even after pretest counseling since decision-making in this population is known to be problematic [25]. How voluntary is acceptance of a test proposed by one's mental health worker? Mental health service staff exercise significant psychological pressure when offering testing and the promise of rapid access to treatment should it be necessary. Even travel vouchers or food snacks may act as an incentive to testing that questions the principle of voluntariness [26]. The extreme poverty of SMI patients means that small compensations can act as inducement that can, depending on person, circumstance, and context, persuade individuals with SMI to disregard any personal risks attached to screening [27].

On the other hand, many SMI patients tend toward stubborn refusal of anything new so that consent, for them, is hard won and requires strong motivation. SMI patients are prone to distrust and may harbor many misconceptions about HIV testing. Some individuals who are suspicious of doctors believe they will be deliberately infected during testing [28]. Because of the high degree of suspicion and mistrust in this population, it is safe to assume that most SMI patients who agree to testing, whether on an opt in or opt out basis, are doing so because the results are important to them.

CONSENT

The principle of informed consent depends on full disclosure of all pertinent information on the part of the responsible staff person, and on the patient's capacity to understand that information and the patient's freedom to choose from available options [29]. Because decisional capacity, the ability to weigh risks against benefits, is impaired in the SMI population, verbal consent to HIV screening may not be considered sufficient. A higher standard for consent should be considered for this population i.e., specific written consent with personal risks and personal benefits of HIV screening explained in full and in written form, with time for patients to think things over and consult with family members should they wish to [30].

It is the responsibility of the staff member to ensure that the patient has the capacity to understand the nature of the test and its possible consequences.

This requires the provision of pre and post test counseling, without which HIV screening could be considered unethical. Pre-test counseling includes discussing the nature of HIV infection, the risk factors involved and methods of prevention. It means explaining the meaning of positive and negative test results and their implications with respect to the need for treatment, the risks of transmission, the emotional impact, and the reactions of others. It also means assessing the patient's personal and social supports and determining whether the patient's emotional strengths are adequate. It requires discussing disclosure of test results to health authorities - requirements vary according to jurisdiction [31] - and family members and ethical obligations (of patient and of health provider) to notify sexual partners and needle sharers. Emotional and mental health consequences of a positive test need to be pre-addressed, as well as the potential reactions of partners and family members. The personal and public health fall out of obtaining early versus late treatment needs also to be thoroughly discussed. Most importantly, patients must be informed that should their choice be to refuse HIV testing, this will not in any way compromise their access to their usual mental health care [29].

Post-test counseling includes informing the patient of the results and the meaning of the test results. If the results are negative, the patient needs to know that this must not be taken as a sign that protection is not necessary but that protective behavior needs to be maintained. Further education about avoiding risks of sexual and injection drug exposures is in order. For patients who test positive, patient and provider must together assess the impact of test results for the patient and family. Treatment options need to be explained and referral made. The disclosure of test results to past and future sexual partners needs to be carefully discussed. It is important to explain to the patient that positive HIV status along with name identification will be provided to health officials. Patients need to know that health records are confidential but may need to be disclosed in certain circumstances, such as subpoenas by the court.

PRIVACY

The issue of privacy is an important one in HIV screening since a breach in confidentiality could potentially result in real or perceived harm. Similar privacy concerns were originally raised with respect to the routine testing of pregnant women but were outweighed by the paramount issue of infant right to health [32-35]. There is legislation relating to confidentiality of HIV tests, reporting requirements, and partner notification that varies with the jurisdiction [36]. The results of the test have to be entered into the medical record and this needs to be explained to patients so that they know what information will be seen should they grant family members or others (Child Protection Agencies for instance) access to their medical files. They must understand the limits of medical file confidentiality, which may differ according to jurisdiction. Patients can ask to see their medical records and make corrections if they spot errors. The mental health team will not reveal the results of the test to others but when screening takes place in a mental health service where members know one another, the word will spread if the patient tells a friend. Patients must be warned about keeping their tests results to themselves and only to disclose to trusted others, otherwise there is no guarantee of privacy.

Equitable Access to Treatment

Currently, the main purpose of HIV testing currently is to obtain rapid access to treatment. There is, in other words, not only a public health but also an individual benefit to knowing one's HIV status. Early access to treatment for the SMI population serves the ethical principle of justice in the delivery of health because it balances the usual lag time before seriously mentally ill populations gain access to treatment. [37,38]. Access is, of course, not sufficient. Patients must be actively encouraged to continue lifelong treatment with drugs that may cause unpleasant side effects [39] and their adherence to treatment needs to be carefully monitored [40], else the whole point of screening is lost.

The Ethics of Partner Notification

Staff providing services to those who test positive for HIV have the added responsibility of urging their patients to disclose their +HIV status to sexual partners and to individuals with whom they share needles or other drug equipment. In nearly two-thirds of US states, individuals who do not disclose their +HIV status and, as a consequence, expose others to HIV, face criminal charges [41]. Staff may also have a duty to warn. An HIV+ patient in a mental health service may have sexual partners and needle sharers who are personally known to staff. They may be fellow service users. This can cause a significant dilemma for the practitioner if the HIV+ patient chooses not to disclose to individuals whom may be at imminent risk. The laws pertaining to duty to warn of +HIV status have to be weighed against the ethical principle of maintaining strict confidentiality. Legislation varies among jurisdictions and, in some, physicians are given a responsibility that differs from that of other health care personnel. In general, the practitioner must try to persuade the +HIV patient to inform his sexual and needle-sharing partners. Sometimes individuals at risk can be warned without revealing the identity of the HIV+ person. If the risk of transmission is high and the patient refuses permission to inform, wide consultation with colleagues and health authorities is warranted, as is extensive documentation in the medical file. The Mental Health Service is under a moral obligation to provide testing and HIV treatment services to individuals who have been infected by their patients even if they are not previous service users. The effectiveness of partner counseling and referral services has been evaluated and, in a review of nine studies, found to be effective. A mean of 67% of identified partners were found and notified of their potential exposure to HIV, and a mean of 63% of those notified were tested (previously known "positives" were not tested). Of those tested, a mean of 20% were found to be HIV positive. There was insufficient evidence as to whether risk behavior was changed or whether transmission was reduced. No substantial harms appeared to result from these procedures [42].

Individual Benefit versus Public Good

It is important to consider and attempt to negotiate a 'balance' of individual and collective interests in the issue of HIV testing [38,43]. Before treatment was available, testing served a public health benefit but the individual being tested was no better off knowing that he/she had been infected. In those days, a change in behavior would benefit others but be of no direct benefit to the patient taking the test. The situation has now markedly changed. HIV testing now has direct benefits because the person who tests positive obtains immediate access to lifesaving treatment. The public benefits as well because early treatment reduces infectivity [44,45].

CONCLUSION

Provider-initiated HIV screening at mental health facilities for the seriously mentally ill is strongly recommended despite concerns about some patients' capacity to fully understand the potential ramifications of a positive test as it pertains to added stigmatization and negative reactions from family and friends. Written consent is recommended for the test. Concerns about undue perceived pressure to comply to screening are probably not warranted. Pre and post test counseling need to be comprehensive so that consent is fully informed and the patient knows how to proceed depending on results of the test. In the case of a positive test, notification of sexual partners and needle-sharing partners may become a responsibility of staff. Treatment needs to be made immediately available and the monitoring of adherence to treatment needs to become an important part of ongoing patient management. HIV testing serves both the individual and the public good.

REFERENCES

[1] Jans L, Stoddard S, Kraus L. *Chartbook on Mental Health and Disability in the United States.* An InfoUse Report. Washington, D.C.: U.S. Department of Education, National Institute on Disability and Rehabilitation Research, 2004.

[2] Meade CS, Sikkema KJ. HIV risk behaviour among adults with severe mental illness: A systematic review. *Clin Psychol Rev* 2005;25:433-457.

[3] McQuillan GM, Kruszon-Moran D, Kottiri BJ, et al. Prevalence of HIV in the US household population: The National Health and Nutrition Examination Surveys, 1988 to 2002. *J Acquir Immune Defic Syndr* 2006;41:651-656.

[4] Blank MB, Himelhoch SS, Balaji AB, et al. A multisite study of the prevalence of HIV with rapid testing in mental health settings. *Am J Public Health* 2014;104:2377-2384.

[5] Walkup JT, Blank MB, Gonzalez JS, et al. The impact of mental health and substance abuse factors on HIV prevention and treatment. *AIDS J Acquired Immune Deficiency Syndromes* 2008; 47:S15-S19.

[6] Branson BM, Handsfield HH, Lampe MA, et al. Revised recommendations for HIV testing of adults, adolescents, and pregnant women in health-care settings. *Morbidity and Mortality Weekly Report.*

Recommendations and Reports/Centers for Disease Control 2006; 55:1–17.

[7] Satriano J, McKinnon K, Adoff S. HIV service provision for people with severe mental illness in outpatient mental health care settings in New York. *J Prev Interv Community* 2007;33:95-108.

[8] Senn TE, Carey MP. HIV testing among individuals with a severe mental illness: Review, suggestions for research, and clinical implications. *Psychol Med* 1009;39:355–363.

[9] Bayer R, Fairchild AL. Changing the paradigm for HIV testing: the end of exceptionalism. *New Engl J Med* 2006;355:647-649.

[10] Cohen SM, Van Handel MM, Branson BM, Hall IH, Hu X, Koenig LJ. Vital Signs: HIV prevention through care and treatment – United States. *Morbidity and Mortality Weekly Report* 2011;60:1618–1623.

[11] Herek GM, Capitanio JP, Widaman KF. Stigma, social risk, and health policy: public attitudes toward HIV surveillance policies and the social construction of illness. *Health Psychol* 2003;22:533–540.

[12] Pierce MW, Maman S, Groves AK, King EJ, Wyckoff SC. Testing public health ethics: why the CDC's HIV screening recommendations may violate the least infringement principle. *J Law Med Ethics* 2011;39: 263–271.

[13] Gielen A, Ghandour R, Burke J, Mahoney P, McDonnell K, O'Campo P. HIV/AIDS and intimate partner violence: Intersecting women's health issues in the United States. *Trauma Violence Abuse* 2007;82:178–198.

[14] Lange T. HIV and civil rights: a report from the frontlines of the HIV/AIDS epidemic. ACLU AIDS Project. November 2003. Available at: http://www.aclu.org/pdfs/hivaids/hiv_civilrights.pdf Accessed Sept. 22, 2014

[15] Schuster MA, Collins R, Cunningham WE, et al. Perceived discrimination in clinical care in a nationally representative sample of HIV infected adults receiving health care. *J Gen Intern Med* 2005;20:807–813.

[16] Kelly C, Alderdice F, Lohan M, Spence D. Creating continuity out of the disruption of a diagnosis of HIV during pregnancy. *J Clin Nursing* 2012;21:1554–1562.

[17] Jürgensen M, Sandøy IF, Michelo C, Fylkesnes K, ZAMACT Study Group. Effects of home-based voluntary counselling and testing on HIV related stigma: findings from a cluster-randomized trial in Zambia. *Soc Sci Med* 2013;81:18-25.

[18] Nuwaha F, Kasasa S, Wana G, Muganzi E, Tumwesigye E. Effect of home-based HIV counselling and testing on stigma and risky sexual behaviours: serial cross-sectional studies in Uganda. *J Int AIDS Soc* 2012;15:17423

[19] Sengupta S, Banks B, Jonas D, Miles MS, Smith GC. HIV interventions to reduce HIV/AIDS stigma: a systematic review. *AIDS Behav* 2011;15: 1075-1087.

[20] O'Grady B, Schüklenk U. Rethinking mandatory HIV testing. *Bioethics* 2009;23(8):ii.

[21] Walkup J, Satriano J, Barry D, Sadler P, Cournos F. HIV testing policy and serious mental illness. *Am J Public Health.* 2002;92:1931–1939.

[22] World Health Organization, UNAIDS. Guidance on Provider-Initiated HIV Testing and Counselling in Health Facilities. Geneva: WHO, 2007. http://who.int/hiv/pub/guidelines/9789241595568_en.pdf Accessed Sept. 22, 2014.

[23] Vernillo A. Routine opt-out HIV testing in dental health care – its implementation and the advancement of public health. *Am J Bioethics* 2011;11:46–48.

[24] Vonn M. British Columbia's 'Seek and Treat' strategy: a cautionary tale on privacy rights and informed consent for HIV testing. *HIV/AIDS Policy Law Rev* 2012;16:15–18.

[25] Cáceda R, Nemeroff CB, Harvey PD. Toward an understanding of decision making in severe mental illness. *J Neuropsychiatry Clin Neurosci* 2014;26:196-213.

[26] Lee R, Cui RR, Muessig KE, Thirumurthy H, Tucker JD. Incentivizing HIV/STI testing: a systematic review of the literature. *AIDS Behav* 2014;18:905–912.

[27] Bentley JP, Thacker PG. The influence of risk and monetary payment on the research participation decision making process. *J Med Ethics* 2006;30:293-298.

[28] Hutchinson AB, Corbie-Smith G, Thomas SB, Mohanon S, del Rio C. Understanding the patient's perspective on rapid and routine HIV testing in an inner-city urgent care center. *AIDS Educ Prev* 2004;16:101–114.

[29] Celada MT, Merchant RC, Waxman MJ, Sherwin AM. An ethical evaluation of the 2006 Centers for Disease Control and Prevention recommendations for HIV testing in health care settings. *Am J Bioethics* 2011;11:31–40.

[30] Njeru MK, Blystad A, Shayo EH, Nyamongo IK, Fylkesnes K. Practicing provider-initiated HIV testing in high prevalence settings:

consent concerns and missed preventive opportunities. *BMC Health* Serv Res 2011;11:87

[31] National HIV/AIDS Clinicians' Consultation Center. Compendium of state HIV testing laws. Available at http://www.nccc.ucsf.edu /consultation_library/state_hiv_testing_laws/ Accessed Sept. 22, 2014.

[32] Fields L, Kaplan C. Opt-out HIV testing: an ethical analysis of women's reproductive rights. *Nurs Ethics* 2011;18:734–742.

[33] Johansson KA, Pedersen KB, Andersson A-K. HIV testing of pregnant women: an ethical analysis. *Dev World Bioethics* 2011;11:109–119.

[34] Seloilwe ES. Commentary on 'Opt-out HIV testing: an ethical analysis of women's reproductive rights'. *Nurs Ethics* 2011;18:743–745.

[35] Wocial LD, Cox EG. An ethical analysis of opt-out HIV screening for pregnant women. *J Obstet Gynecol Neonatal Nurs* 2013;42:485-491.

[36] Hanssens C. Legal and ethical implications of opt-out HIV testing. *Clin Infectious Dis* 2007;45:S232–S239

[37] Frohlich KL, Potvin L. The inequality paradox: the population approach and vulnerable populations. *Am J Public Health.* 2008;98:216–221.

[38] Knight R, Shoveller J, Greyson D, Kerr T, Gilbert M, Shannon K. Advancing population and public health ethics regarding HIV testing: a scoping review. *Critical Public Health,* 2014;24:283–295.

[39] Abers MS, Shandera WX, Kass JS. Neurological and psychiatric adverse effects of antiretroviral drugs. *CNS Drugs* 2014;28:131-145.

[40] Joska JA, Obayemi Jr A, Cararra H, Sorsdahl H. Severe mental illness and retention in anti-retroviral care: A retrospective study. *AIDS Behav* 2014;18:1492–1500.

[41] Lehman JS, Carr MH, Nichol AJ, Ruisanchez A, Knight DW, Langford AE, Gray SC, Mermin JH. Prevalence and public health implications of state laws that criminalize potential HIV exposure in the United States. *AIDS Behav* 2014;18:997–1006

[42] Hogben M, McNally T, McPheeters M, Hutchinson AB. The effectiveness of HIV partner counseling and referral services in increasing identification of HIV-positive individuals – a selective review. *Am J Prev Med* 2007;33(Suppl 2):S89–S100.

[43] Daniels N. Equity and population health: toward a broader bioethics agenda. *Hastings Center Rep* 2006;36: 22–35.

[44] Bayer R, Edingtom C. HIV testing, human rights, and global AIDS policy: exceptionalism and its discontents. *J Health Polit Policy Law* 2009; 34:301–323.

[45] Dawson A. Public health ethics and the justification of HIV screening. *Am J Bioethics* 2011; 2011;11:48–49.

In: Patient Rights
Editor: Jenna Pope
ISBN: 978-1-63482-136-0

Chapter 7

TRUTH-TELLING, BEST INTERESTS, AND AUTONOMY

Kam-Yuen Cheng[*]
Centennial College, Pokfulam, Hong Kong

ABSTRACT

Physicians generally accept two major reasons for nontruthful disclosure of information to patients even when the patients can make autonomous decisions: promoting the patients' best interests and preserving their autonomy. If physicians deceive or withhold information from such patients based on the first reason, the physicians act from paternalism. However, autonomous individuals are in the best position to determine their best interests. The manner in which patients understand their best interests may differ from the physician's perceptions; therefore, respecting patients' autonomy, rather than paternalistic practice, is the best way to promote patients' best interests. Nontruthful disclosure of information can be justified only when truth-telling will cause patients to lose their ability to make decisions reflecting their long-term values, i.e., only when truth-telling will compromise patients' autonomy. In general, paternalism is justified only when patients' autonomy has already been or is going to be compromised.

[*] Corresponding author: Kam-Yuen Cheng. Centennial College, 3 Wah Lam Path, Pokfulam, HK. E-mail address: kycheng@hkuspace.hku.hk.

INTRODUCTION

The practice of truth-telling or honesty is a presupposition in the doctor-patient relationship. Many people, both doctors and patients, however, think that patients' right to the truth (including diagnosis, prognosis, and treatment risks[1]) can be violated in some exceptional situations. In the clinical context, nontruthful disclosure of information includes providing false or misleading information, or simply withholding information that is necessary for making autonomous health-care-related decisions[2]. Physicians generally accept two major reasons against truth-telling in this context: 1) promoting patients' best interests[3] and 2) preserving patients' autonomy. Other reasons include maintaining the ward's social order and the fact that medical evidence is based on probabilities and thus medical results are never certain[4]. The last two reasons are obviously unjustified. Regarding maintaining the ward's social order, on the one hand, if the objective is to let health professionals work efficiently or to protect them from discomfort, non-truthful disclosure of information will violate patients' best interests and violate their right to informed consent and thereby their right of autonomy. On the other hand, if the objective is to promote patients' interests, this objective has the identical reason to the first, which I will discuss in detail. Regarding the probabilistic nature of medical evidence, patients can simply be informed about the probabilities on which their diagnoses or prognoses are made. Therefore, I will focus on the first two reasons.

I. PROMOTING BEST INTERESTS

The reason that people think nontruthful disclosure of information can promote patients' best interests in some situations (e.g., in cases of terminal ill patients or patients who are sole survivors of an accident) is that truthful disclosure will cause distress and anxiety that will affect the patients' physical and psychological well-being.

---

[1] Oakley (2007) argues that the surgical risk (mortality rate) of particular surgeons should also be disclosed to patients.

[2] Dying patients may want to finish the "unfinished business" of their lives. Hence, letting them know their imminent death will help them decide when to do such things. Although such decisions are not medical decisions, I count them as "health-care-related decisions."

[3] I include preserving hope in this category.

[4] Some people also appeal to cultural differences. But the fact that medical paternalism is commonly practiced in a culture does not mean that its practice is justified in that culture.

Nonetheless, Buchanan (1978) points out that we must not only consider the harms involved in informing; rather, nontruthful disclosure is justified only when its harm is smaller than the harm of truth-telling (378). Such comparative judgments require doctors to know not only their patients' current physical and psychological conditions, but also the patients' personalities and life experiences.

Doctors should also include in their judgment the possible harm caused to their patients if the patients discover the nontruthful practice. In addition, Higgs (2009) reminds us that "if [patients] do not have the information on which to base a choice, or even a realization that a choice is necessary at all, it seems hard not to see this in itself as a major harm" (523). More accurately, what Higgs is saying is that nontruthful disclosure of information will violate patients' right of autonomy.

Assuming that, from the physician's perspective, the harm of informing is larger than that of deception or withholding information in a particular situation, we still need to ask whether this can justify the violation of the patient's right of autonomy.

According to the US President's 1982 "Commission for the Study of Ethical Problems in Medicine, and Biomedical and Behavioral Research":

> When the conflicts that arise between a competent patient's self-determination and his or her apparent well-being remain unresolved after adequate deliberation, a competent patient's self-determination is and usually should be given greater weight than other people's view on that individual's well-being. (26)

That is, patients' autonomy should be valued higher than their physician's understanding of their best interests. The reason behind this claim is that competent, or more correctly, autonomous patients are held to be in the best position to determine their best interests. In an example of diabetes patients, Stewart and DeMarco (2004) demonstrate that a physician's preferred level of treatment is often different from a patient's because the physician's preferred level is usually higher than the level that maximizes the patent's marginal health-care-related interests. In the case of terminally ill patients, the physician may think that maximizing the span of a painless life is in the patient's best interest, whereas the patient may regard a life without meaning as torture[5].

---

[5] Of course, the physician should try to come to a consensus with the patient in terms of treatment level, but such consensus presupposes truthful disclosure.

In the case of euthanasia, if the family of a comatose patient requests the physician to withdraw a respirator to let the patient die, what the physician should consider first is not what he or she believes to be the patient's best interests, but what the patient *would do* if he or she were competent and autonomous. Hence, the patient's best interests as understood by the physician cannot trump the patient's right of autonomy. Paternalism is only justified when the patient's autonomy has already been or is going to be compromised.

II. PERSERVING AUTONOMY

Now I will discuss preserving patients' autonomy as a reason for nontruthful disclosure of information. Suppose that a physician has evidence, not just a belief, that truthful disclosure will bring emotional trauma to a patient resulting in his or her loss of autonomy. Such a situation would justify deception or withholding information because autonomous consent cannot be obtained anyway. However, as Buchanan points out, such evidence involves psychiatric generalizations, which ordinary physicians may not be in a position to recognize and assess (379). Therefore, in order to acquire such evidence, they will probably need to consult psychiatrists or psychologists.

We should also note that there is a distinction between autonomy and competence. Autonomy presupposes a higher level of rationality than competence. A patient is competent as long as he or she has the basic ability to understand and to communicate, and does not make gross logical mistakes. However, a patient's choice is nonautonomous if it is *largely* inconsistent with his or her long-term values. Clarke (2001) indicates that medical decisions are different from decisions in other areas. As he points out, regarding areas outside medicine, "If someone is competent to make decisions to consent, then they are generally regarded as entitled to do so in any way in which they see fit" (181). By contrast, informed consent is required for an autonomous consent in medicine. This requirement exists to make sure that the decision reflects, or is authenticated by, the patient's long-term values. Nonetheless, not every choice that is inconsistent with one's long-term values should be considered nonautonomous. For example, smokers and skydivers make autonomous decisions in choosing their habits and sports even though they have long life as their long-term values. Their behaviors, unlike Jehovah's Witnesses' refusing of blood transfusion, do not constitute a large threat to their long-term values. In other words, smokers and skydivers' irrationality is just not high enough to render their behaviors nonautonomous.

Consequently, when physicians have evidence that truthful disclosure will cause patients so much distress or anxiety that they will likely make decisions that are a larger threat to their long-term values, deception or withholding information is justified in this case. However, having such evidence requires physicians to know their patients well.

CONCLUSION

Many ethicists[6] argue that promoting patients' best interests can justify nontruthful disclosure of information even when the patients can make autonomous decisions. I have argued against these ethicists. Autonomous patients are in the best position to determine their best interests. Respecting their autonomy is the best way to promote their best interests as they understand themselves. The only reason that can justify nontruthful disclosure is to preserve patients' autonomy. In order to obtain evidence showing that deception or withholding information does preserve patients' autonomy, general physicians will need to consult psychiatrists or psychologists and to know the long-term values of their patients. Of course, patients may choose not to know the truth. Therefore, in order to respect patients' autonomy, a physician can simply ask them whether they would like to have all of the information the physician has about them as soon as possible. The expression "all of the information" here means the information without which a rational person may make a different health-care-related decision.

Sharing information with the patient as soon as possible does not mean divulging information in a single interview. The study of Davis et al. (2002) shows that patients can retain only about 50% of information during a single interview (quoted in Richard et al. 2010: 356). As Richard at el. points out, "If the objective is to have the patient understand the situation, the necessary discussion should be limited to what the patient is able to understand and remember" (2010: 357). Therefore, divulging information in a series of sessions is necessary and should not be counted as withholding information.

In fact, physicians can fully respect patients' autonomy only if they can understand the patients well. This, in turn, requires a continuous dialogue between the patients and the physicians.

[6] Examples include Sokol (2007), Richard et al. (2010), and Pergert and Lützén (2012).

REFERENCES

Buchanan, Allen. 1978. "Medical Paternalism." *Philosophy and Public Affairs* 7: 370-390.

Clarke, Steve. 2001. "Informed Consent in Medicine in Comparison with Consent in Other Areas of Human Activity." *Southern Journal of Philosophy* 39: 169-187.

Davis, T., M. Williams, E. Marin, et al. 2002. "Heath Literacy and Cancer Communication." *CA: A Cancer Journal for Clinicians* 52: 134-149.

Higgs, Roger. 2009. "Truth-telling." In: *A Companion to Bioethics*, ed. Kuhse and Singer. Malden: Wiley-Blackwell.

Oakley, Justin. 2007. "Patients and Disclosure of Surgical Risk." In: *Principles of Health Care Ethics*, ed. Ashcroft et al. West Sussex: John Wiley and Sons.

Pergert, Pernilla and Kim Lützén. 2012. "Balancing Truth-telling in the Preservation of Hope: A Relational Ethics Approach." *Nursing Ethics* 19: 21-29.

Richard, C., Y. Lajeunesse and M. Lussier. 2010. "Therapeutic Privilege: Between the Ethics of Lying and the Practice of Truth." *Journal of Medical Ethics* 36: 353-357.

Sokol, Daniel. 2007. "Can Deceiving Patients be Morally Acceptable?" *British Medical Journal* 334: 984-986.

Stewart, Douglas and Joseph DeMarco. 2004. "An Economic Theory of Patient Decision-Making." *Journal of Bioethical Inquiry* 2: 153-164.

United States. 1982. *President's Commission for the Study of Ethical Problems in Medicine and Biomedical and Behavioral Research: Making Health Care Decisions*. Washington: GPO.

In: Patient Rights
Editor: Jenna Pope
ISBN: 978-1-63482-136-0

Chapter 8

PROBLEM IN ETHICS FOR MEDICAL PUBLICATION: BRIEF REVIEW AND CASES FROM THAILAND

***Somsri Wiwanitkit*[1] *and Viroj Wiwanitkit*[1,2,3,4,5]**

[1] Wiwanitkit House, Bangkhae, Bangkok, Thailand
[2] Hainan Medical University, China
[3] Faculty of Medicine, University of Nis, Serbia
[4] Joseph Ayobabalola University, Nigeria
[5] Surin Rajabhat University, Surin, Thailand

ABSTRACT

Medical publication is a common kind of literature in medical journals and books. Similar to any other kinds of science, the ethical problems in medical publication can be seen and it is an interesting issue in journalism. The misconducts in medical publication is of concern and the management is required. Here, the authors brief review and discussed on examples from Thailand.

INTRODUCTION

Medical publication is a common kind of literature in medical journals and books. Similar to any other kinds of science, the ethical problems in medical publication can be seen and it is an interesting issue in journalism. The misconducts in medical publication is of concern and the management is required. The three main kinds of misconducts include plagiarism, falsification and fabrication. Here, the authors brief review and discussed on examples from Thailand.

THE PRESENT SITUATION IN THAILAND

As a developing countries with a number of ethical problem, the problems of misconducts in medical publication is very common in Thailand. Hundreds of misconducts can be identified. The problem seems complicated and there is no proper management of the misconducts. Lohsirwat and Lohsiriwat noted that "the system of handling research misconduct is still lacking [1]." Some seniors or administrators who perform misconduct still get no punishment. Some get promotion to be higher rank based on their problematic non ethical publications. It is a long way but should be promoted to upgrade the standard for the Thai to avoid misconduct in medical publication [2].

CASE EXAMPLES

Here, the authors would like to introduce some interesting examples from Thailand. All cases are real things but the names will be blinded for privacy reason.

1) "I miscarry the file and have it published in the textbook. So I will cut the pages of the chapter that is a plagiarism"

   The case started when an associate professor in a Clinical Pathology Department found that a chapter in a published textbook of the department is totally from her previously paper document for teaching medical students. The author of that problematic chapter is the head of the department. This associate professor decided to report this problem to the dean of the Faculty of Medicine and the dean called the head of department for clarification. The head of department said that she was innocent. She said "I miscarry the file and have it published in the textbook. So I will cut the pages of the chapter that is a plagiarism". She also noted that she had conflict with the associate professor who reported the problem and thought that that associate professor was bad that used this story to harm her. She cried when she reported to the dean. Finally, the dean did nothing and notified the associate professor not to speak out this story to protect the fame of the faculty. Finally, the head of the department get higher rank to become a professor in Clinical Pathology.

2) "I am an assistant dean of Faculty of Medicine who corresponds to manage misconduct in the faculty. I get award as national young eminent scientist. But I have a self-plagiarism publication."

The case is of an assistant dean of Faculty of Medicine who corresponds to manage misconduct in the faculty. This assistant dean in research affair gets award as national young eminent scientist. He tried to blame many ones in the faculty and accuses them for having misconduct. But this assistant dean was finally diagnosed to have a self-plagiarism publication. The problem was reported to the faculty but no punishment was done. In addition, an unexpected event occurred. The faculty administrator tries to force the one who report the problem, who is a junior in the faculty, to resign from the faculty. Also, the dean of the faculty tries to write the confident letter to the journal asking the manager of the journal to support that the actual plagiarism is innocent and the manager of the journal accept to unethically help.

3) "I am a medical professor with more than 10 plagiarisms publication. When the problem is detected, I change my institute to another institute and have my name and surname change."

The case is of a medical professor with more than 10 plagiarisms publication. When the problem was detected, this professor changed the institute to another institute and had my name and surname changed. He became the dean in the new institute. However, after nationwide talk and rumors on this story, he had to resign from the position of the dean but still be a senior consultant in that institute.

4) "I am the national eminent scientist with many international publications on infectious diseases (eg. hepatitis, influenza, etc.) I am the board of many journals. When I was young I plagiarize the others' article, using the figure and textual contents with translation and non - proper citation. I presently promote practice against misconduct of the others"

The case is of a national eminent scientist with many international publications on infectious diseases (eg. hepatitis, influenza, etc.) He acts as the board of many journals and have high H-index. He presently promotes practice against misconduct of the others and he is the ethical committee of many institutes. However, he was diagnosed to have at least on plagiarized work that he performed since he was still a young scientist. He plagiarized the others' article published in Singapore, using figure and translated textual contents without proper citation. The institute of this medical professor does nothing for this problem.

5) "Since this young researcher gets many publications, I and my colleague fell jealous and try every way to get rid of this researcher. I have a good plan, have a worker in the university to send a problematic file from the young researcher's computer and plays a drama to force that young researcher to accept that he performs a plagiarism on my name"

This is the most complicated case. The story is of a young researcher who gets many publications. Due to rapid academic growth of this junior research, he becomes the target of jealousness by many other senior practitioners. There are many attempts to get rid of this young scientist. Finally, a tricky plan was generated. The bad senior team including bad senior professor and administrator in the institute had a lay worker to use the personal computer of the junior researcher when he was absent. That computer was used to send a file of an article with the name of senior professor in the bad team to a medical journal. That file is problematic and totally plagiarized from others. Finally, the medical journal detected the problem and reported the case to the institute. The senior medical professor refused the problem and had the local IT police to trace the file of plagiarized article and found that the file was from the computer of the junior researcher. The junior researched was accused for causing the problem and forced to accept the punishment. The junior researcher can do nothing. This is a bad drama that should never exist in medical society.

Conclusion

Styles of misconduct in medical publication in Thailand are very complex. Many examples are extremely interesting. The important notification that there is no good system for management of the problem, both punishment of the senior who performs misconduct and help support the young researcher who witness and report the problem [3 – 5].

REFERENCES

[1] Lohsiriwat V, Lohsiriwat S. Fraud and deceit in published medical *J Med Assoc Thai.* 2007 Oct;90(10):2238-43.
[2] Wiwanitkit V. How to avoid plagiarism. *Ann Biomed Eng*. 2013 Jan;41(1):3.
[3] Wiwanitkit V. Plagiarism, management *Saudi J Anaesth.* 2013 Apr;7(2):223.
[4] Wiwanitkit V. Simultaneous submission, duplicate publication, self-plagiarism and the proper management *J Minim Access Surg*. 2014 Jan;10(1):51.
[5] Wiwanitkit S, Wiwanitkit V. Plagiarism, self-plagiarism and scientific misconduct: preventive and correction action. *Vaccine.* 2013 Apr 3;31(14):1765.

In: Patient Rights
Editor: Jenna Pope

ISBN: 978-1-63482-136-0

Chapter 9

PATIENTS' RIGHTS IN INDIA: DO THEY ASSURE EMPOWERMENT?

***Ravindra B. Ghooi*[*1] *and Shailesh R. Deshpande*[2#]**
[1]Scientia Clinical Services, Pune, India
[2]Chellaram Diabetes Institute, Pune, India

ABSTRACT

The patient is the central figure in any healthcare system. In fact, she is the reason the system exists. In India, though the entire health care system has evolved around the patient, it is, strangely, the healer who is looked upon as the patron of the system. The doctor is positioned at the top of the social hierarchy while the patient is at the bottom, though the latter pays for everything. In the entire process, patients have few rights, and even those are limited to what the doctors deign to grant them. Doctors ensure that their authority never gets diluted. In case of disputes, medical colleagues support the doctor and not the patient. The patient is a helpless pawn in the game played by doctors, hospitals, laboratories and drug companies.

---

* Ravindra B. Ghooi, Director, Scientia Clinical Services, G801 Rohan Nilay, Aundh, Pune 411007; Tel: +912025882021, Mobile +919922918967; E Mail: Ravindra.ghooi@gmail.com

Shailesh R. Deshpande, Head, Education and Training, Chellaram Diabetes Institute, 1st Floor, Lalani Quantum, Pune-Bangalore National Highway 4, Bavdhan (Budruk), Pune, Maharashtra 411021.

Patients' rights are meant to protect them from these situations and any form of financial impropriety violates these rights. Unfortunately, financial impropriety in the medical world is a pervasive phenomenon, seen more often in developing countries where it is rampant throughout the hierarchy. This prevents the patients from having access to quality medical care. In India, the existing patients' rights provide no protection since the charter of rights is designed not to empower the patient, but to keep him in the power of the doctor.

The average Indian survives many battles against health hazards caused by low quality water supply, poor sanitation, low standards of public health, high morbidity and mortality as well as indifference of doctors and administrators in the healthcare system. This leaves the citizens caught between a highly inefficient public health system and a largely unregulated and exploitive private health system. The physician, who is the final link to the patient, has the power to protect the patient, but more often than not, stands as a mute spectator. Patients here require more rights, especially those that will protect them against financial exploitation. They should also have the right to decide how they are treated in the terminal stages and should have the option to put in place directives that are legal and binding on families and attending physicians.

INTRODUCTION

The treatment meted out to the weaker sections of society reflects the progress of civilization. In a highly civilized society, the individual, whether able-bodied or disabled, is treated fairly and with respect, so no special rules need be prescribed for such a society. In other societies, people with physical, mental or social disabilities have a lower status and quality of life and, therefore, need protection. Countries are ranked on the basis of the Human Development Index. People living in countries with lower Human Development Index [1] need to be provided with rights if they are to live with liberty and equality. In 2014, India is ranked at 135 of 187 countries and grouped with countries with a medium Human Development Index.

Rights organizations have defined what rights an individual has, yet very few deal with the individual's right to health. [2] The Universal Declaration of Human Rights is an excellent document, articles of which find support in the constitutions of many free countries, but it does not specify the rights of patients. [3] Associations of physicians world over have prepared charters of patients' rights and so have some consumer protection organizations. The rights granted to patients are mainly non-financial and demand no sacrifices from other stakeholders in healthcare. None of the charters that list patients' rights grants them any financial power. As a result, patients continue to pay more for services that are progressively worsening.

The doctor is a key person in the healthcare system. She wields tremendous influence and has the power to ensure good service to the patients. Unfortunately, the doctor is often hand in glove with those who exploit the patients. If the doctors really took their roles seriously and followed their ethical codes meticulously even a poor orphan would be secure in the system. A few decades ago, the medical profession was considered 'noble'. Today not even doctors can honestly describe themselves so. The doctor-patient relationship has deteriorated steadily. In many developed countries, patients are suing doctors for actual and imagined wrongs, and doctors are investing heavily in protecting themselves through insurance. In this struggle, both parties, i.e., doctors and patients, are the losers and the only winners are lawyers and the insurance companies.

The healthcare system consists of a large number of other stakeholders; the industry that manufactures and markets medical products, the retailers who sell these products, hospitals that provide medical support, the laboratories where investigations are done and so on. These stakeholders vigorously defend their profit margins, passing on every cost to the end user, the patient. Governments are also involved in this; they tax every stakeholder and the burden gets passed on to the patient. The price of every medicine or medical device snowballs as it moves down the supply chain and the patient pays a huge price for something that otherwise would cost a fraction.

Like many other interactions, the physician-patient interaction must be viewed as a partnership for promoting health. In some countries, such partnerships ensure mutual benefits and cost savings [4] but such evidence is lacking in India. [5] In any partnership, both the parties must profit, but if one profits at the cost of the other, it is exploitation and not a partnership. Sadly, this is true for doctor-patient relationships in developing countries today. [6] Worldwide, this relationship is accepted to be a fiduciary one, where one party (patient) places his/her complete confidence and trust in the other party (physician). Though this is not formally established, the doctor is bound by moral and ethical codes to provide a standard of care. [7]

Despite many instances of unethical practices on the part of physicians coming out in the open, very few are actually investigated and punished. Courts have upheld the role of the physician as that of a service provider and have held him/her responsible for providing a standard of care, when that care is provided at cost. [8] Legal procedures in developing countries, however, are so slow that getting justice from the legal system is but a dream.

The rights of the patients and the duties of the physician are corollaries to each other. As stated earlier, rights of the patients have been defined by bodies that represent doctors. There are different models of physician-patient relationships which are reflected in charters of patients' rights prepared in countries where these models dominate. [9]

In India, patients' rights are defined by the Medical Council of India as a part of the Code of Medical Ethics. [10] In chapter 2, the code defines the obligations of physicians to their patients, many of which are conveniently forgotten by doctors.

The rights mentioned in this document stem from the duties of the physician and are not patient centric. [11] It is amply clear that in the obligations to the patients, doctors are not obliged to provide their patients the best medical service for the fees that they receive. This has been left out either by error or by design. A charter of patients' rights is also prepared by the Consumer Guidance Society of India. This is more detailed and is supported by the MCI code of conduct. However, these rights are basic and do not provide any real protection to the patients.

In India, it is more relevant to study the rights listed by the Consumer Guidance Society of India and check their consonance with Code of Ethical Regulations (COER) of the Medical Council of India. The number in the brackets refers to the particular article of the COER of the MCI regarding this aspect.

1. *You have a right to be told all the facts about your illness, to have your medical records explained to you and to be made aware of risks and side effects, if any, of the treatment prescribed for you. Do not hesitate to question your doctor about any of these aspects*

The Code of Ethical Regulations does not address this issue, but enjoins all physicians to give factual information to patients and their relatives (2.3). It is accepted that most patients do not have the basic knowledge of human physiology to understand the disease they suffer from, nonetheless it is the duty of the doctor to explain the ailment to the patient to the best of his ability. Often, patients' relatives or friends could be in a better position to understand the medical situation, and hence, patients should be encouraged to bring along someone who has a better understanding. Inclusion of this aspect in the COER would make doctors more conscientious about imparting information to the patients and their relatives. Granted that in a crowded public hospital the doctors too are pressed for time, but this could be done by junior doctors or trained nurses too.

2. *When you are undergoing a physical examination, you have a right to be handled with consideration and due regard for your modesty*

This issue is not addressed in the COER, but is generally practiced in the country. However the possibility of examination in open wards does exist in overcrowded public hospitals. One of the authors (SRD) has been witness to a scene in a large public hospital where a gynecologist was repeatedly slapping a woman in labor on her thighs and verbally abusing her for delaying the process of labor. It is another thing that the patient ultimately decided to give back and kicked him in his face!

3. *You have a right to know your doctor's qualifications. If you cannot evaluate them yourself, do not hesitate to ask someone who can*

The COER requires that doctors provide this information without being asked (1.4.2). Some related issues need to be clarified here. In India, there are a large number of doctors practicing modern medicine without being qualified to do so. There are three types of unqualified people who practice modern medicine. First are the frauds (quacks) that have no qualifications at all. Second group is those with qualifications not recognized by the governments. The last group comprises those who hold qualifications in alternative medical systems but practice modern medicine. This observation is validated by an earlier study by the Centre for Economic and Social Studies. [12]

Some states in India have granted permission to the last group of practitioners under the assumption that a partly qualified doctor is better than having no doctor at all. Allowing Complementary Alternative Medicine (CAM) practitioners to practice modern medicine as a mechanism to tide over the crisis of doctors in rural areas may be justifiable. However, not creating conditions for these practitioners to practice their own science deprives patients of the choice for CAM. The option then is of going to spas or other such centers that are prohibitively expensive, thus negating the idea that CAM are people-centric therapies. Many of the junior doctors in large hospitals in cities are CAM graduates, but practice modern medicine.

4. *You have a right to complete confidentiality regarding your illness*

The COER supports this right, and it is respected in private practice and hospitals. How confidential this information is in the public set up is really unknown (2.2). In national programs addressing tuberculosis and HIV/AIDS, diseases prone to stigmatization, safeguards exist for ensuring confidentiality of the patient. For other conditions, mechanisms for confidentiality may not be robust.

5. *If you are doubtful about the treatment prescribed and especially an operation suggested, you have a right to get a second opinion from any specialist*

The COER supports this, but asks physicians not to let differences of opinion come out in the open. (3.4.2) Thus if a physician has given a wrong advice, his peers are not likely to contradict it, at least openly. The system of clinical audits is rudimentary and non-binding in India. This makes it very difficult for a patient to take legal recourse against bad medicine, since the medical fraternity tends to protect their own.

6. *You have a right to be told in advance what an operation is for and the possible risks involved. If this is not possible because of your being unconscious or for some other reasons, your nearest relatives must be told before they consent to the operation*

The COER, while supporting this, suggests the use of a consent form to be signed before any surgery. (7.16) Many times, alternatives to the operation are not given. For instance, sterilizations are still preferred in the public sector when ample options like oral contraceptives and intrauterine devices are available. Many hysterectomies are fraudulent, carried out by unscrupulous doctors to "provide comfort" to the women and also as a means of family planning.

In a recent tragedy in Indian State of Chhattisgarh, a tubectomy camp left 19 women dead. In the past, similar tragedies have occurred in camps, where those in-charge try to establish records of performing a large number of procedures in a given time. There could be other examples like the conventional appendectomies and tonsillectomies or the modern-day laser and cosmetic surgeries, often carried out in place of better and safer alternative forms of medical therapies.

7. *If you are to be discharged or moved to another hospital, you have a right to be informed in advance and to make your own choice of hospital or nursing home, in consultation with the doctor*

This issue is not addressed in the MCI's COER. Most hospitals are not keen to transfer their patient to another hospital. In the public healthcare system, the healthcare facilities are ill-equipped to manage the patient. Hence, the patient is referred to a higher center, when she could have been managed at a lower level facility. Serious or "difficult" patients and medico-legal cases are avoided by private facilities and referred to government hospitals. Worse, private hospitals sometimes, "experiment" with treatments, causing a lot of unnecessary expenditure to patients and then refer them to other hospitals, claiming inability to manage the condition despite the best of efforts. This is also observed with many cancer patients.

8. *You have a right to get your case papers upon request*

The COER acknowledges this right and puts a time line of 72 hours to respond to it (1.3.2). However, this may also turn into a frustrating experience for patients and their relatives as many hospitals delay the requests citing heavy workloads.

A reading of this bill of rights makes it clear that patients are granted rights which are only due to them. As consumers, they would have far more clout, but doctors do not want patients to be given the status of consumers, since then they will be held accountable for the services provided. Despite the fact that legal system of India is notoriously slow, the courts have repeatedly come out in favor of patients. In a landmark case, the Supreme Court held that the Consumer Protection Act of 1986 (CPA) was applicable to the medical profession, over the objections of the profession. [13] However, how the CPA is going to be applied to CAM practitioners is difficult to guess.

It must be remembered that a patient's fight with the doctor or the hospital is in the David versus Goliath category. The patient is a single individual who takes on an established organization like a hospital or the medical fraternity. Powers of the two adversaries, whether financial or otherwise, are grossly unequal. Though the COER mandates that physicians "should expose, without fear or favor, incompetent or corrupt, dishonest or unethical conduct on part of members of the profession" (COER 1.7), a doctor rarely opines against a colleague.

The slow pace of the judicial system affects both sides; it may take the courts up to 15 years to award a settlement in a case of medical negligence [14] and up to 25 years to acquit a doctor in another. [15] There isn't any data available on how many complaints were received by the MCI or the State Medical Councils over a period of time regarding professional malpractice, how many were acted upon, what actions were taken, the follow-up, etc. Ideally, this data should be available on their websites; it would give transparency to the functioning of these bodies.

While the Medical Council of India is an arbitrator in disputes between patients and their doctors, corruption at the highest level of the MCI has been a matter of concern. [16] In May 2010, the then President of the MCI, Dr. Ketan Desai, was arrested following the recovery of large amounts of unaccounted precious metals and cash from his residence. He was also alleged to own over 400 properties across the country. It was further alleged that this fortune was amassed by collecting bribes for granting recognition to private medical colleges. He was booked under the *Prevention of Corruption Act* and his license to practice medicine, revoked. [17] Dr. Desai was later set free under mysterious circumstances. He then served the World Medical Association as its President during the years 2011-12. [18]

Since the Consumer Protection Act (CPA) brought healthcare under its purview, members of the medical profession have protested against medical practice being equated with a service and patients being treated as consumers. [19,20] The courts make a distinction between private and public medical services. Patients in the private sector are treated as consumers while those in public sector are not. This is not in the interest of those seeking medical treatment from public hospitals. [21]

The plans of the government to protect patients suing the doctors or hospitals under the CPA are greatly supported by the courts, which is the only succor to people. The treatment meted out to patients in India and in many developing countries is pathetic.

The rights given to them are not respected; at times patients aren't even treated like humans but rather like commodities. Nowhere is this more apparent than in the recent Chhattisgarh tragedy highlighted above. However, it cannot be disputed that the patient has rights as a human being, some of which are corollaries to other rights and some, implied. Consider the following:

1. The patient has a right to receive the best and most appropriate treatment whether medical, surgical or otherwise

In a number of situations in India, this right is violated. The manufacture, sale and prescription of spurious, substandard medicines, [22] avoidable surgeries, [23, 24] and needless hospitalization are all examples. A book devoted to avoidable heart surgeries has been published in an Indian language in 2013. [25] A number of serious scientific articles have challenged the need for bypass surgeries in a large number of patients [26] and a number of fictional narratives have touched upon this topic. [27] In all these situations, the patient is forced to undergo a procedure which could have been avoided. In most cases, it is the doctor who impresses on the patient the need to undergo the procedure in the face of which, the patient has no options.

A corollary to this right is that the patient should be informed of other forms of treatment available for the particular ailment. By this, it is meant that available alternative therapies should be detailed. [28] Despite the fact that the doctor may or may not have faith in those systems, a patient certainly has a right to choose them. [29] In conditions where drug therapy, surgery, radiation or palliation are the alternatives, they should be discussed as dispassionately as possible. For instance, studies have demonstrated that there is little to choose between different modes of adjuvant therapy to surgery in squamous cell carcinoma of the esophagus. [30] It is recognized that in case of cancer, each specialist advises the treatment which is in his branch of specialization, giving evidence to the saying '*to a man with a hammer, everything looks like a nail*' (Mark Twain).

Another corollary to this right is the right to protection against over medication. Patients should be informed that in certain diseases like hypertension and diabetes, medication is not the only resort. Emphasis on diet and lifestyle is essential, though the doctor might find it easier to prescribe some drugs than imparting this important information.

Proper treatment or 'best treatment' also refers to quality of care, which means minimum standards of care should be provided. While standard treatment protocols and evidence-based medicine are the norm in the developed world, these concepts are in their infancy in India. Therefore, there is wide variation in disease management from doctor to doctor. This results in a lot of difficulties for the patient, including doctor-hopping, increased costs of care and a loss of confidence in the medical profession. In the case of antibiotics, with an increasing resistance to many frontline antibiotics, there is a danger to the society at large.

2. The patient has the right to receive the most economical treatment suited for his/her disease

Patients very often are prescribed expensive brands of drugs, though the COER of the MCI requires doctors to prescribe generic drugs only. A survey of 990 prescriptions showed that 90% of prescriptions were for branded medicines, clearly showing that the MCI's Code of Ethics is not followed by doctors. [31]

As a result of past patent laws, there are a large number of brands of a single generic drug with varying prices. Doctors raise the bogey of quality whenever the branded versus generic drugs debate surfaces, [32] but fail to explain their preference for the most expensive brands when more affordable ones are available in the market. They also fail to appreciate that the growth of Indian Pharmaceutical Industry is mainly due to manufacture and export of generic drugs. [33] As it is, the variation in drug prices in India is so wide that patients end up paying way above the cost of the drug. Table 1 lists a few common drugs and the variations in prices of their brands.

Table 1. Comparison of the most economical vs. the least economical brands of select medicines available in the Indian market

No.	Generic Name	Most Economical	Least Economical	High/ Low Ratio
1	Ampicillin 500 mg	Rs. 3.60	Rs. 7.45	2.07
2	Glimepiride 1 mg	Rs. 0.95	Rs. 5.50	5.78
3	Amlodipine 5 mg	Rs. 1.00	Rs. 8.25	8.25
4	Metformin 500 mg	Rs.0.60	Rs. 2.20	3.67
5	Tamoxifen 10 mg	Rs. 1.90	Rs. 3.30	1.73
6	Carbamazepine 200 mg	Rs. 1.00	Rs. 2.20	2.20

* Source: www.medlineindia.com database.

The only justification for choosing a brand is bioavailability, but authentic data on bioavailability is rarely available in India and the choice is based on factors not connected with the quality of the product. The role of the pharmaceutical industry in influencing prescribing habits has been discussed at length. The conclusions are not very complimentary for the medical profession. [34] Gifts given by the pharmaceutical industry are known to affect prescribing habits, irrespective of the value of the gift. [35]

In India generic drugs are often manufactured by the same companies that manufacture branded drugs. A study of generic drugs in comparison with branded drugs manufactured by the same organization revealed that there was no difference in the quality of the five commonly used drugs. [36] Due to differences in pricing of branded versus generic drugs, the patient gets significant economic relief when generics are prescribed. [37]

As a corollary to this right, the patient should be allowed to voice his/her concerns about the cost of therapy and the doctor must consider prescribing the least expensive therapy that is available without compromising quality of treatment. Cost-minimization analysis is often undertaken by hospitals [38] and the benefit of that should be extended to patients who are paying for it. Pharmaco-economic studies should be undertaken when two therapies have equivalent effect or when drugs from different sources are being compared. [39]

Most private hospitals have a retail drug store attached to them. This store is usually owned and operated by the hospital management or a party closely related to it. Most in-patients are encouraged, sometimes even forced to buy their medical requirements from this store when the same drugs or equipment are available at much lower rates outside in the city. [40]

Medical practice involves a lot of pecuniary deals between doctors and other stakeholders, such as the pharmaceutical industry, hospitals, laboratories etc. A doctor may prescribe a drug because the industry gives him an incentive. These paybacks are common in all countries, but the COER specifically warns against such practices (COER 6.4.1). [41]

Alternately, a doctor may patronize a laboratory for the commissions he receives. From the point of view of the practitioner, these kind of gains have become acceptable over a period of time. As Asawari Sant puts it, *"a wrong done over and over again by a large number of people, and highly educated people at that, soon becomes the order of the day.* [42] Doctors should remember that their patronage to someone comes at an added cost to their patients.

The provision to display the rates of services at the hospitals in the proposed Maharashtra Clinical Establishments Act is a bone of contention. "Every patient is different, so how can rates be standardized" is the refrain from the establishments. However, in most developed countries, this has been achieved, so it should be possible in India too.

3. Patients have the right to refuse futile repeat testing and to pay for it

A more insidious practice adopted by hospitals is insisting that all investigations be done at their own laboratories. This practice possibly began when it was found that test reports from other laboratories were not trustworthy enough to base clinical decisions upon. [43] Today it is a method of ensuring that the laboratory attached to the hospital remains profitable.

Van Walraven and Raymond, in 2003, commented that the problem of repeat testing has not been adequately studied, [44] and there is a scarcity of reports from India about the extent of this problem. However, doctors have complained that laboratories offer payments for referring patients to them for diagnostic testing. [45] Elsewhere, there is a concerted effort to reduce such testing, [46] but in India, since it is done at the behest of hospitals, it is doubtful if any such efforts will be made.

There are in India a number of NABL (National Accreditation Board for Testing and Calibration Laboratories) accredited laboratories. Tests done at such centers need not be repeated at hospitals. If they are, it is clearly a violation of patients' rights and makes a joke of the accreditation. [47] Accreditation by a national body implies that the laboratory tests samples accurately. Repeating tests done at accredited laboratories suggest that the repetition is being done for malafide reasons.

4. Patients have a right to be treated with dignity

Just because a person has fallen ill, he or she should not be denied basic courtesy. Elderly patients are often addressed by their first names (which is not culturally acceptable in India) since they are sick. [48] Healthcare professionals can practice patient-centered care by treating patients with respect, giving honest information, making them feel valued as persons and by inviting them to take part in all decisions about their daily life and care. [49] A colleague once confided to the authors that when he was ill, he was addressed by his first name and not by his honorific 'Dr'. The argument was that he had earned this title and his illness could not take away this achievement. Many doctors have experienced this, and when they do so, they come out against it, but one wonders how many of them address their own patients with due respect.

One way of respecting the patient is by attending to her as promptly as possible. It is common in India for doctors to meet their patients three or four hours after the time of appointment. This is not restricted to free treatment in public hospitals, it is equally common in highly expensive private set-ups. Influential patients are given priority over other patients, irrespective of the fact that they both are paying patients. Unfortunately, doctors have fallen into a habit of keeping patients waiting. One of us (RBG) was once invited to a meeting by a practicing doctor, since the doctor needed help. However, she could not get over her habit of keeping people waiting and did not turn up even two hours after the decided time. On repeated questioning the receptionist gave a curt reply - 'The doctor will come shortly, she has asked you to wait'. When talking to patients, words like 'please' or 'sorry' are rarely used. The COER of MCI does speak about the need to be punctual and polite, but like many other ethical regulations, doctors have given it a miss.

In a recent incident, the wife of a medical colleague was undergoing chemotherapy at a leading private hospital. Since she was covered by insurance, the doctor in charge of chemotherapy, refused to remove the catheters (a central line was being used) till the bills were signed by the representatives of the insurer. When the colleague objected, he was brashly told that this is the way the patient will be treated and it matters little if the complainant was a medical professional. When this issue was brought to the notice of the hospital management, the concerned doctor apologized, but gave the excuse that she did not know 'that the patient was so well connected'! In India, it appears that empathy and decent behavior are only meant for 'well connected' patients.

Consequently, apart from dignity, patients should be treated without discrimination of any kind, be it gender, race, religion or socio-economic status.

5. The right to ask for futile treatment to be withheld or stopped

The lives of patients are often prolonged by therapy and measures that do nothing except prolong life. Therapies or measures that do not add value to life, or make a patient more comfortable towards the end, should be considered futile. Such therapy should be discontinued at the earliest. This is not mercy killing or euthanasia, it is humane medicine. [50] Similarly, a dying patient should be given adequate analgesia, sedation to reduce the distress as a part of palliative medicine. [51]

The corollary to this right would be alleviating the pain of a suffering patient. For instance, palliative care is the right of patients in terminal stages of cancer and should be provided to them. This is essential since oncologists do not refer patients for palliative care, though it is available freely in some Indian cities.

6. The patient's values and beliefs should be respected.

India is a vastly diverse country. Patients come from varied socio-cultural backgrounds, with differing choices and opinions that should be respected by the healthcare providers. Their preferences in the process of care should be accommodated as far as possible.

"The health of my patient will be my first consideration," states the Declaration of Geneva, [52] while the International Code of Medical Ethics declares that, "A physician shall act in the patient's best interest when providing medical care." [53] While registering as a physician with the MCI in India, a doctor signs a declaration including statements which bind her to the aforesaid principles. Somewhere down the line, the focus on the patient and her benefits gets lost and replaced with extraneous concerns. As a result, the physician, who is the most important protector of the patients, stands by silently when the patients' rights are violated and they are cheated by the industry, trade, hospitals and laboratories.

There is a need to reaffirm rights of the patients, not by professional bodies representing doctors or the industry, but by patients' bodies and these rights must include one for protection against exploitation. The doctor is the greatest protector of patients. If they are vigilant and honest, if they really accept that the health of their patient is their first responsibility, then patients would not require a charter of rights. The need for patients' rights has come up because the patient is being exploited by the healthcare system. Many doctors join others in exploiting the patients, and the good ones, unfortunately, stand by as mute spectators.

The Declaration of Helsinki, the Belmont Report and numerous other ethical guidelines have granted protection to subjects of medical research. However, very little has been done to protect ordinary patients who outnumber research subjects. Can the World Medical Assembly or the World Health Organization take up this task that has been pending for long?

Over a hundred years ago, Sir Robert Hutchinson wrote a poem that is remembered even today. [54] He prayed for the humane practice of medicine for which there is a real need today. It is surprising that Sir Robert predicted in 1897, what is wrong with the practice of medicine today. His words below echo what is largely the voice of millions of citizens under duress from the healthcare system today.

'From inability to let well alone
From too much zeal for the new and contempt for what is old
From putting knowledge before wisdom, science before art, and
Cleverness before common sense;
From treating patients as cases;
And from making the cure of the disease more grievous than the
Endurance of the same, Good Lord, deliver us.' – *Sir Robert Hutchison.*

Conflict of Interest:

The authors have no conflict of interest to declare.

Declaration:

The views expressed herein reflect those of the authors and may not be attributed to the organizations they represent.

REFERENCES

[1] United Nations Development Program. Human Development Report 2014. Available at: http://hdr.undp.org/sites/default/files/hdr14-report-en-1.pdf

[2] Hall, MJ. Advancing Climate Justice and the Right to Health through Procedural Rights. *Health and Human Rights Journal* 2014; 16(1): 8-18.

[3] United Nations. The Universal Declaration of Human Rights. Available at: http://www.un.org/en/documents/udhr/index.shtml#a14

[4] Pham HH, Alexander G, O'Malley AS. Physician's consideration of patients' out-of-pocket costs in making common clinical decisions. *Arch Intern Med* 2007; 167(7):663-8.

[5] Berger D. Corruption ruins doctor patient relationship in India. *BMJ* 2014; 348:g3169-70.

[6] Gopichandran V. Doctor-patient relationship-from blind faith to strategic trust. BMJ 2014 Blog. Available at: http://blogs.bmj.com/bmj/2014/02/04/vijayaprasad-gopichandran-the-doctor-patient-relationship-from-blind-faith-to-strategic-trust/

[7] Physician Patient Relationship. Law & Legal Definition. Available at:http://definitions.uslegal.com/p/physician-patient-relationship/

[8] K. Ganesh. Patient-doctor relationship: Changing perspectives and medical litigation. Indian J Urol 2009; 25(3):356-60.

[9] WHO Patients' Rights. World Health Organization, 2014. Available at http://www.who.int/genomics/public/patientrights/en/

[10] Medical Council of India. Code of Ethics Regulations, 2002 (Amended up to December 2010). Available at: http://www.mciindia.org/RulesandRegulations/CodeofMedicalEthicsRegulations2002.aspx

[11] Ghooi RB, Deshpande SR. Patients' rights in India: an ethical perspective. *Ind J Med Ethics* 2012; 9:277-81.

[12] Narayana KV. The unqualified medical practitioners. Working Paper No. 70. 2006 Available at: http://www.cess.ac.in/cesshome/wp%5Cwp-70.pdf

[13] Debbarma J, Gupta N, Aggarwal NK. Consumer Protection Act – Blessing or curse to Medical Profession? *Delhi Psychiatry Journal* 2009; 12(2):302-5.

[14] Nischal PM Supreme Court orders highest ever compensation in case of medical negligence. *Natl Med J. India* 2013; 26(6):380-1.

[15] Johari V. Professional misconduct or criminal negligence: when does the balance tilt? *Ind J. Med. Ethics* 2014; 11 (2):117-20.

[16] Mahajan V. White coated corruption. *Ind. J. Med. Ethics* 2013; 7(1):18-20.

[17] Pandya S. The Medical Council of India: need for a total overhaul. Ind J Med Ethics 2014; 11(2):68-71.

[18] Bhan A. Globalizing the rot within? *Ind. J. Med. Ethics* 2010; 7(2):124.

[19] Keaney M, Are patients really consumers? Intern J Soc Econ 1999; 26(5):695-707.

[20] Bakshi SM. A study of patient satisfaction at a tertiary care hospital in Hyderabad, India. *World Hosp Health Serv* 2013; 49(2):26-9.

[21] Agrawal AD, Banerjee A. Free medical care and consumer protection. *Indian J. Med. Ethics* 2011; 8(4):240-2.

[22] Srinivasan S. The "spurious drugs" gene and its pervasiveness. *Indian J. Med. Ethics* 2010; 7(3):136-9.

[23] Mark DB, Knight JD, Velazquez EJ, Howlett JG, Spertus JA, Djokovic LT, et al. Quality of life and economic outcomes with surgical ventricular reconstruction in ischemic heart failure: results from the Surgical Treatment for Ischemic Heart Failure trial. *Am. Heart J.* 2009; 157(5):837-44.

[24] Coulm B, Blondel B, Alexander S, Boulvain M, Le Ray C. Potential avoidability of planned cesarean sections in a French national database. *Acta Obstet Gynecol Scand* 2014; 93(9):905-12.

[25] Choudhury BR. *Heart Mafia*. Faridabad: World Records University; 2013.

[26] Ornish D. Avoiding revascularization with lifestyle changes: The Multicenter Lifestyle Demonstration Project. *Am. J. Cardiol.* 1998; 82(10B):72T-76T.

[27] Klaidman S. *Coronary: A true story of medicine gone awry*. New York: Scribner; 2008.

[28] Kelner M, Wellman B. Health care and consumer choice: Medical and alternative therapies. *Soc. Sci. Med* 1997;45(2):203-12.
[29] Chan A, Wong A. Is combined chemotherapy and radiation therapy equally effective as surgical resection in localized esophageal carcinoma? *Int. J. Radiat. Oncol* 1999; 45(2):265-70.
[30] Prise EL, Etienne PL, Meunier B, Maddern G, Hassel MB, Gedouin D. A randomized study of chemotherapy, radiation therapy, and surgery versus surgery for localized squamous cell carcinoma of the esophagus. *Cancer* 1994; 73:1779-84.
[31] Patel V, Vaidya R, Naik D, Borker P. Irrational drug use in India: A prescription survey from Goa. *J. Postgrad Med.* 2005; 51(1):9-12.
[32] Paul Y. Why should I not prescribe branded drugs? *Indian J. Med. Ethics* 2012; 9(2):138.
[33] Greene W. The Emergence of India's Pharmaceutical Industry and Implications for the U.S. Generic Drug Market. US International Trade Commission, 2007; Office of Economics Working Paper No. 2007-05-A. Available at: www.usitc.gov/publications/332/EC200705A.pdfc
[34] Wazana A. Physicians and the Pharmaceutical Industry – Is a Gift Ever Just a Gift? JAMA 2000; 283(3):373-80.
[35] Katz D, Caplan AL, Merz JF. All Gifts Large and Small: Toward an Understanding of the Ethics of Pharmaceutical Industry Gift-Giving. *Am. J. Bioeth* 2010; 10(10):11-7.
[36] Singal GL, Nanda A, Kotwani A. A comparative evaluation of price and quality of some branded versus branded-generic medicines of the same manufacturer in India. *Indian J. Pharmacol* 2011; 43(2):131-6.
[37] Heaney DC, Sander JW. Antiepileptic drugs: generic versus branded treatments. *Lancet Neurol* 2007; 6(5):465-8.
[38] Dasta JF, Kane-Gill SL, Pencina M, Shehabi Y, Bokesch PM, Wisemandle W, Riker RR. A cost-minimization analysis of dexmedetomidine compared with midazolam for long-term sedation in the intensive care unit. *Crit. Care Med.* 2010; 38(2):497-503.
[39] Newby D, Hill S. Use of pharmacoeconomics in prescribing research. Part 2: cost-minimization analysis – when are two therapies equal? *J. Clin. Pharm. Ther* 2003; 28:145-50.
[40] Godwin SK, Varatharajan D. Drug price differentials across different retail market Settings-An analysis of retail prices of 12 commonly used drugs. *Health Administrator* 2006; 19(1):41-7.
[41] Thomas G. Gifts to doctors, scientific information and the credibility gap in the Medical Council of India. *Indian J. Med. Ethics* 2010; 7(2):68-9.

[42] Sant A. Problems with private pathology practice. Issues Med Ethics 2003; 11(3):99.

[43] Branger PJ, Van Oers RJM, Van Der Wouden JC, Van Der Lei J. Laboratory services utilization: a survey of repeat investigations in ambulatory care. *Neth J. Med* 1995; 47(5):208-13.

[44] Van Walraven C, Raymond M. Population-based Study of Repeat Laboratory Testing. *Clin. Chem.* 2003; 49(12):1997-2005.

[45] Jesani A. Professional codes, dual loyalties and the spotlight on corruption. *Ind. J. Med. Ethics* 2014; 11(3):134-6.

[46] Young DW. Improving laboratory usage: a review. *Postgrad Med. J.* 1988; 64:283-9.

[47] Wadhwa V, Rai S, Thukral T, Chopra M. Laboratory quality management system: Road to accreditation and beyond. *Indian J. Med. Microbiol.* 2012; 30:131-40.

[48] Rajgopal MR. Disease, dignity and palliative care. *Indian J. Palliat Care* 2010; 16(2):59-60.

[49] Kvåle, K, Bondevik, M. What is important for patient centred care? A qualitative study about the perceptions of patients with cancer. *Scand. J. Caring Sci.* 2008; 22:582-9.

[50] Saunders C. Euthanasia-definition, dangers and alternatives. *Ann. Acad. Med. Singapore* 1994; 23(2):300-3.

[51] Enck RE. Drug-induced terminal sedation for symptom control. *Am. J. Hosp. Palliat Care* 1991; 8(5):3-5.

[52] World Medical Association. The Declaration of Geneva. Available at: http://www.wma.net/en/30publications/10policies/g1/

[53] World Medical Association. International Code of Medical Ethics. Available at: http://www.wma.net/en/30publications/10policies/c8/

[54] Shanker RP. Sir Robert Hutchison's Petition and the Medical Humanities. *Int. J. Med. Educ.* 2010; 1:2-4.

INDEX

A

B

C

D

E

I

J

L

M

N

O

P

T

U

V

W

X